Scars After Surgeries in the Abdominal Area

Springer Nature More Media App

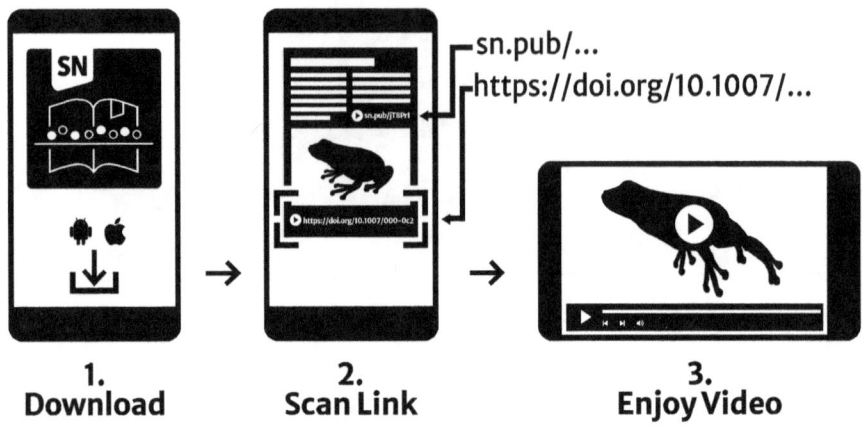

Support: customerservice@springernature.com

Michaela Liedler

Scars After Surgeries in the Abdominal Area

Self-Help with the Liedler-Concept

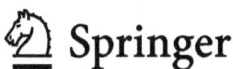

Michaela Liedler
Vienna, Austria

This work contains media enhancements, which are displayed with a "play" icon. Material in the print book can be viewed on a mobile device by downloading the Springer Nature "More Media" app available in the major app stores. The media enhancements in the online version of the work can be accessed directly by authorized users.

ISBN 978-3-662-71376-1   ISBN 978-3-662-71377-8 (eBook)
https://doi.org/10.1007/978-3-662-71377-8

Translation from the German language edition: "Narben nach Operationen im Bauchraum" by Michaela Liedler, © Der/die Herausgeber bzw. der/die Autor(en), exklusiv lizenziert an Springer-Verlag GmbH, DE, ein Teil von Springer Nature 2024. Published by Springer Berlin Heidelberg. All Rights Reserved.

This book is a translation of the original German edition "Narben nach Operationen im Bauchraum" by Michaela Liedler, published by Springer-Verlag GmbH, DE in 2024. The translation was done with the help of an artificial intelligence machine translation tool. A subsequent human revision was done primarily in terms of content, so that the book will read stylistically differently from a conventional translation. Springer Nature works continuously to further the development of tools for the production of books and on the related technologies to support the authors.

© The Editor(s) (if applicable) and The Author(s), under exclusive license to Springer-Verlag GmbH, DE, part of Springer Nature 2025

This work is subject to copyright. All rights are solely and exclusively licensed by the Publisher, whether the whole or part of the material is concerned, specifically the rights of translation, reprinting, reuse of illustrations, recitation, broadcasting, reproduction on microfilms or in any other physical way, and transmission or information storage and retrieval, electronic adaptation, computer software, or by similar or dissimilar methodology now known or hereafter developed.
The use of general descriptive names, registered names, trademarks, service marks, etc. in this publication does not imply, even in the absence of a specific statement, that such names are exempt from the relevant protective laws and regulations and therefore free for general use.
The publisher, the authors and the editors are safe to assume that the advice and information in this book are believed to be true and accurate at the date of publication. Neither the publisher nor the authors or the editors give a warranty, expressed or implied, with respect to the material contained herein or for any errors or omissions that may have been made. The publisher remains neutral with regard to jurisdictional claims in published maps and institutional affiliations.

This Springer imprint is published by the registered company Springer-Verlag GmbH, DE, part of Springer Nature.
The registered company address is: Heidelberger Platz 3, 14197 Berlin, Germany

If disposing of this product, please recycle the paper.

Contents

1 From Layman to Expert in Terms of Scars—Adhesions in the Tissue and Adhesions in the Abdominal Cavity — 1
  1.1 The Effects of Surgery — 1
  1.2 Treatment Fundamentals — 4
  1.3 Sliding Mechanisms in the Body—Mobility of Connective Tissue — 17
  1.4 Wound Healing — 18
  References — 24

2 Consequences of Surgeries — 29
  2.1 Why do Adhesions Occur Particularly during Surgeries? — 29
  2.2 Small Skin Incision (Laparoscopy) versus Large Skin Incision (Laparotomy) — 30
  2.3 Effects of Scars and Adhesions on the Body (see Fig. 2.3) — 32
  2.4 The Factor of Time—What Happens in the Body when the Scars are Old? — 40
  2.5 Tissue—Mechanical Influenceability of Adhesions in the Tissue and Adhesions in the Abdominal Cavity — 43
  2.6 Scars as Part of Life History (Understanding—Physically and Mentally) — 45
  References — 49

Contents

3 The Basics of the Liedler Concept (LK)   51
    3.1   Therapeutic Approach—Idea and Goal of LK Self-Exercises   52
    3.2   When to Delay Self-Exercises   53
    3.3   Setting the Right Focus and Using Two Basic Principles   54
    3.4   The Scoop Grip   61
    3.5   Identifying Restrictions with the Scar Check of the Liedler Concept   63
    3.6   The Levels of Scar Treatment   68
    3.7   Delineation from Other Scar Treatment Concepts   70
    3.8   The Topic of Pain in the Liedler Concept   70
    3.9   How the Timing of the Operation Affects Therapy   75
    References   79

4 Practice—HandsOn   81
    4.1   Practical Recommendations and Self-Exercises   81

5 Questions and Answers   109
    5.1   Questions about the Scar   109
    5.2   Questions about the LK Self-Exercises—Application   113
    5.3   Preparation for an Operation, Support of Wound Healing and Therapy   116

1

From Layman to Expert in Terms of Scars—Adhesions in the Tissue and Adhesions in the Abdominal Cavity

1.1 The Effects of Surgery

Surgeries are part of everyday medical practice. The scars left behind not only feel new and initially uncomfortable on the outside. A surgery also leaves its mark beneath the scar in the deeper layers of the body. During the healing process, adhesions and growths form in the deeper tissue layers. In the abdominal cavity, these are medically referred to as peritoneal adhesions. If one compares the after-effects of a surgery metaphorically with an iceberg, the scar visible on the surface corresponds to the tip of the iceberg, while the adhesions represent the large invisible volume of the iceberg (see Fig. 1.1). Especially in the context of laparoscopy, where the surgery is performed using an abdominal mirror without a large abdominal incision, the incisions in the body are minimal when viewed from the outside. However, it is easily overlooked that the size of the wound in the abdominal cavity and under the skin, where the actual surgery took place, is much larger.

Even though the body's own wound healing generally aims to reconnect and heal the tissue layers well after a surgical intervention, excessive tension can occur. This is perceived as a more or less distinct feeling of burning, tingling, itching, or pulling. There can also be a feeling that the affected area is cut off from the body, or simply a discomfort associated with this area.

Adhesions inside the body are unfortunately difficult for doctors to diagnose. Therefore, they often remain both undetected and untreated, hidden beneath the surface of the skin. As a result, many pain symptoms associated

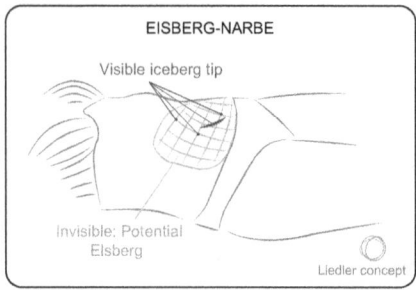 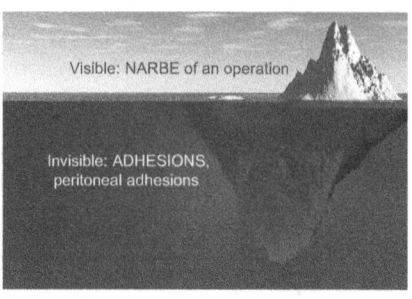

Fig. 1.1 Scar as the tip of the iceberg and adhesions as the body of the iceberg. (© 2022 Liedler-Concept/iStock: Getty Images)

with these adhesions, such as chronic tension, back pain, spinal complaints, pain during intercourse, infertility, etc., are often dismissed as psychosomatic or as a psychological problem, and the patients' own perception is portrayed as wrong and impossible.

Scientific studies on manual therapy forms and manual treatment possibilities in this regard are unfortunately scarce. Therefore, these therapy forms are rarely recommended by doctors. Nevertheless, practice shows that there are various good possibilities to treat the entire iceberg. A real noticeable improvement and thus a significant relief as well as a new body feeling can be achieved in many ways. The Liedler Concept is a very effective way in this context, as it includes both the surface and the body depth in the therapy. The focus of the Liedler Concept is on adhesions in the tissue and in the abdominal cavity, and above all the sustainable treatment.

According to studies, adhesions after surgery occur in 50 to 99% of all surgeries in the abdominal cavity (Liedler 2020). The problem is therefore known in medicine, but is difficult to visualize beyond surgical assessment. Therefore, adhesions in the abdominal cavity and in the deep tissue layers often remain undetected.

The effects of adhesions in the tissue and in the abdominal cavity are rarely discussed or treated due to difficult diagnostic representation or complex subsequent possibilities for remedy. The causal connection between adhesions and chronic pain is considered by the treating physicians far too rarely. These adhesions often contribute to chronic pain conditions in the rest of the body, such as shoulder and neck pain, chronic back pain, bladder problems, superficial breathing, tension states, etc. Creating a general awareness of these potential effects on the body can be essential for recognizing necessary treatment. Based on the following list of relevant and common symptoms after surgery, you may already be able to draw your own initial conclusions (see Overview).

This is exactly where the Liedler Concept (LK) comes in. With the help of a manual scar test specifically developed within the framework of the Liedler Concept, it makes actual restrictions in the tissue and their effects on large movement chains in the body visible and palpable. The subsequent treatment options and LK self-applications can quickly and effectively influence and resolve these restrictions. Those who prefer to be treated rather than take matters into their own hands are recommended to the therapists trained according to the Liedler Concept. They are listed on narbenzentrum.at as "certified LK therapists". In parallel, there is the professional book "Peritoneal Adhesions—Fascial Treatment according to the Liedler Concept", which was published by Springer Verlag in 2020, for professional colleagues.

Apart from professional manual therapy, the Liedler Concept is also highly effective in self-treatment. Every affected person can use it to find out for themselves whether there is currently a restricted mobility of the body system, triggered by the scar and the associated deeper adhesions. At the same time, they can then actively contribute to the restoration of their body comfort.

List of relevant and common symptoms that occur after surgeries due to adhesions and scar tissue

- Shortness of breath
- Breathing problems (only superficial, no deep abdominal breathing possible anymore)
- Temporomandibular joint complaints, reduced mouth opening, cracking of the temporomandibular joints
- Persistent tension in shoulders and shoulder girdle
- Back pain in the thoracic spine
- Neck tension
- Headaches
- Back pain (lumbar spine), the feeling of "breaking off and not being able to move anymore"
- Frequent, sudden twisting of the spine
- Pain and blockages of the pelvic joints (sacroiliac joints—SIJ)
- Sciatica pain
- Stiff pelvis, reduced pelvic mobility
- Hip pain
- Knee pain (usually increased on the side of the surgery)
- Occurrence of painful, difficult to influence muscle hardening and muscular pain points in the body (trigger points)
- Sleeping on the stomach no longer possible

- Bladder problems (pressure on the bladder, incontinence, "smaller bladder", needing to go to the toilet frequently, complete emptying of the bladder not possible)
- Menstrual pain, PMS
- Pain during sexual intercourse
- Recurring, pulling pain during movement and strain

Specifically after surgeries in the upper thorax or neck area (e.g. thyroid)

- Neck tension
- Back pain in the thoracic spine
- Tension between the shoulder blades and in the chest area
- Temporomandibular joint complaints—cracking
- Difficulty lifting arm (usually one-sided)

Specifically after joint surgeries

- Feeling of stiffness in the surgical area or/and the adjacent joints
- Persistent or recurring swelling of the scar area
- Lymphatic drainage disorders
- Pulling pain during movement and strain
- Faster fatigue of the scar area under strain

The Liedler Concept allows to specifically, clearly, and effectively make existing adhesions and scar tissue noticeable as well as their effects on the rest of the body visible. At the same time, it provides the tools to quickly and sustainably change and dissolve these.

1.2 Treatment Fundamentals

Scars, adhesions, and agglutinations are terms that are often used in a similar context. However, it is of great importance for therapy after surgery to know that these structures per se differ from each other, i.e., they are constructed differently and can affect the body system differently. For the duration and the estimation of the success of therapy, it makes a big difference whether the treatment mainly involves scar tissue, adhesions in the tissue, or agglutinations in the abdominal cavity, as each of these structures reacts differently in the treatment process. Especially deep agglutinations in the abdominal cavity and adhesions in the deep tissue layers often remain undetected. The following section is intended to help understand these structures and the structure of the tissue in the body better and to develop a sense for the changes in one's own body and/or to be able to name them. Many of you will already know the symptoms and in the best case then know exactly what it is that feels different than before the operation.

1.2.1 Definitions: Scar, Adhesion, Agglutination in the Abdominal Cavity

In the literature, but also in practice, the terms "scar", "adhesion in the tissue", and "agglutination in the abdominal cavity" are used in similar contexts again and again. Therefore, the terms will be briefly illustrated more precisely, defined, and their effects described in the following.

1.2.1.1 Scar

A scar primarily refers to the superficially visible skin and primarily serves to quickly and efficiently cover any damage in and on the body, thereby closing a wound. Scar tissue is always formed in the same way, regardless of the type of injured tissue. This applies to the skin, muscles, or tendons. The maximum strength of scar tissue varies from person to person and depends on various factors, including the size and depth of the original injury, the way the wound was treated, and other individual health factors. However, scar tissue usually reaches about 80% of its maximum strength after about 3 months to a year after the injury or surgery (Guimberteau and Armstrong 2016).

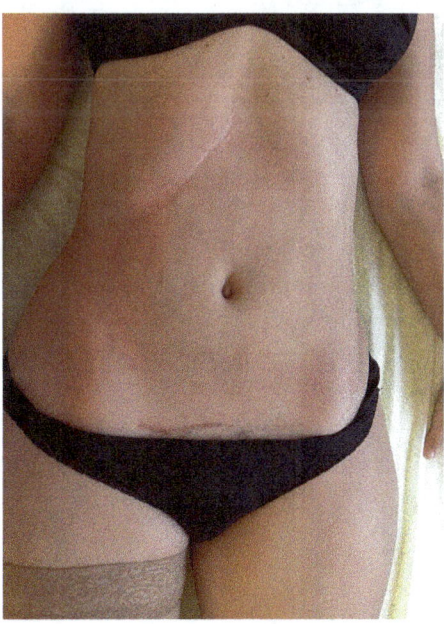

In the formation of scar tissue, unorganized and thickened tissue fibers made of collagen are deposited, which results in the loss of the sliding of the tissue layers and thus parts of the mobility in this area (Asmussen and Söllner 2010). For the body to maintain its health, it must be supple, able to move easily inside and out. This allows it to adapt effectively and flexibly (Bouffard et al. 2008; Fourie 2014; Guimberteau and Armstrong 2016). Depending on the size of the wound, the destruction of the tissue, and possible complications during the healing process, different variations in the quality of the scar tissue arise (Guimberteau and Armstrong 2016; Stöckl 2019).

Scars are classified according to their shape and appearance into normal inconspicuous (physiological) and conspicuous (pathological) scars. In addition, they are characterized as flat, retracted, atrophied (healed below skin level), or raised. A well-healed scar is soft and movable, white, can be touched, moved, and lifted relaxed, and is otherwise inconspicuous.

All other types of scars can have different effects on the body and negatively affect the quality of life of the affected person at different levels (Bordoni et al. 2023).

Under certain circumstances, the scarred skin changes and retractions, a tension, a nerve severance, or the ingrowth of free nerve endings into the scar can lead to an irritation of the scar tissue or to a persistent irritation in the affected area. All of this promotes permanent local inflammatory processes and prevents the healing process from being completed. Thus, the scar can remain sensitized and conspicuous (Bordoni et al. 2023; Guimberteau and Armstrong 2016; Stöckl 2019).

An impairment of the sliding layers of the affected and surrounding connective tissue can then lead to restrictions of the motor function and the development of compensation patterns (Fourie 2014). An excessive proliferation of scar tissue is referred to as hypertrophic or keloid scar and divided. While the excessive scar usually subsides on its own over the years and adapts to the surrounding skin level, the underlying persistent processes in keloid scars are not yet clarified. Different genetic and cellular causes as well as altered, continuous inflammatory processes seem to lead to a constant exaggerated overproduction of scar tissue and hypersensitization of the associated nervous system. As a result, keloid scars often remain (very) painful and prove to be protracted and difficult to treat (Bordoni et al. 2023). The goal is that through treatment with the Liedler Concept, the tissue can become as supple as possible again and the body can calm and regulate excessive reactions and inflammations (as in the adhesions section).

1.2.1.2 Fascial Adhesion—Tissue Adhesion

Tissue Adhesion vs. Healthy Connective Tissue

While normal healthy tissue shows a fine movable, elastic, and flexible spider web structure, adhesions are recognized by dense, immovable fiber strands in the tissue (Fig. 1.2).

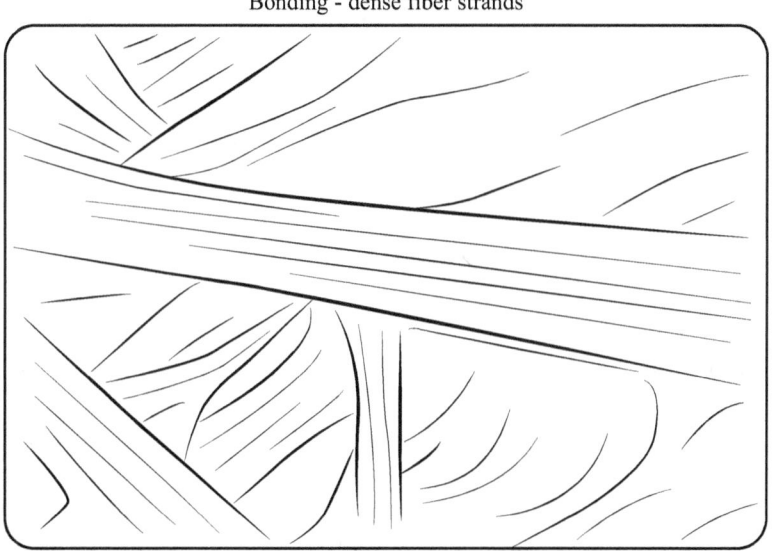

Bonding - dense fiber strands

> **Why is the scar area often perceived as more sensitive or numb than before?**
> Nerve fibers, which inform us about pain in the tissue, usually lie inactive in loose tissue. When these free nerve endings now grow into the dense tissue connections and adhesions, they become irritated, the scar area becomes more sensitive than before and can possibly also trigger pain. The goal is that the suppleness in the tissue is restored through treatment with the Liedler Concept and thus the pain sensitivity normalizes and disappears.

In medical and common everyday language, scar tissue and adhesions are often equated. However, it is important to distinguish precisely, because adhesions represent a complication of scarring. The good thing is that adhesions can be well influenced in manual therapy and are open to change or for manual therapy. Healthy tissue is characterized by a fine, chaotic

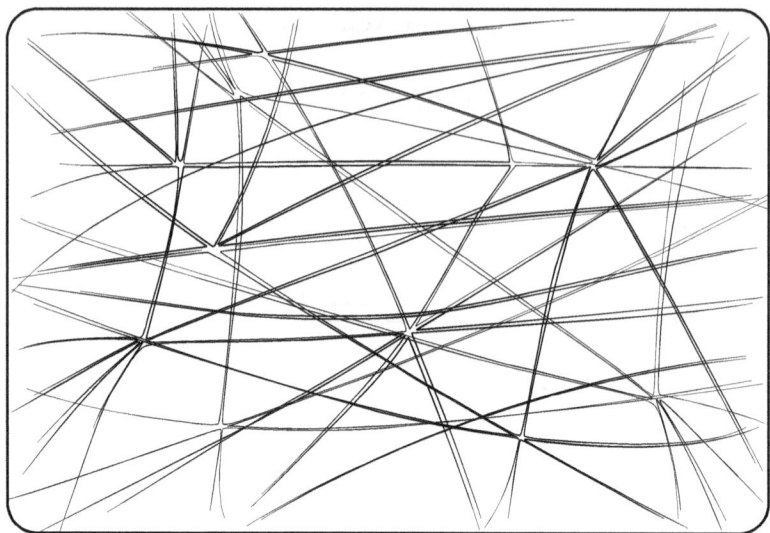

Fig. 1.2 Healthy Connective Tissue

network of thin, spider web-like collagen fibers, which represent the prerequisites for flexibility and functionality. Depending on the location and position, the tissue, also known as fascia, is structured accordingly. Superficial fascial layers support the mobility of the skin and have a protective function by absorbing force and pressure. Deep, more powerful fascial layers lie on the muscles and support them in translating force into movement, efficiently transmitting and distributing it. Tensile stresses and pressure loads thus determine how the tissue fiber network is formed to enable the corresponding movements. In the case of greater loads, tissue injuries or traumas, the body is able to reinforce the fibers via additional connections and to network them more closely (Ingber 2008a; Schleip 2003a, b, Van den Berg 2014a,b).

Adhesions are recognized by inflexible tissue strands in all types and forms, as densifications of connective tissue, which can form in the most varied structures and layers both superficially and in depth. Stiffness and immobility without functional purpose are the result. Irritations caused by tension pulls, triggered by adhesions and reaching deep into the tissue, as well as the lack of normal and easy mobility of the tissue can impair the supply of the tissue during wound healing and also prevent the completion of repair mechanisms (Guimberteau and Armstrong 2016). Pain fibers are also found here, which grow into the adhesions and thickened fibers instead of lying loose and free in the connective tissue. The consequence is that muscle activity and movements cause tensions that act on the adhesions, thereby triggering pain stimuli (Stöckl 2019) and can lead to irritations, compensation patterns and chronic pain conditions.

1.2.1.3 Peritoneal Adhesions—Adhesions in the Abdominal Cavity

During surgery deep is intervened into the body. This means specifically that during surgery in the abdominal cavity, first the skin as well as the superficial and deep tissue layers are cut open, then by tearing or cutting the abdominal membrane sac (medically: Peritoneum), in which the organs lie, is opened, to reach the place where the actual operation takes place. From the outside, it will not be recognizable how large the wound actually is, which must heal invisibly in the body or in the abdominal cavity afterwards. During this wound healing, adhesions in the abdominal cavity are formed (see Fig. 1.3) (Bordoni et al. 2023; Cheong et al. 2001; Pados et al. 2010).

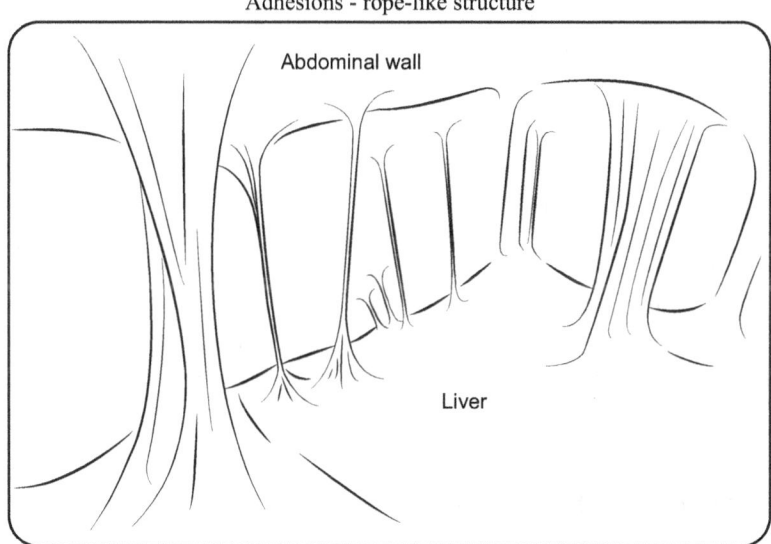

Adhesions in the abdominal cavity describe extra tissue connections between organs and/or the abdominal membrane sac, which are not originally laid out. The main cause for the formation of adhesions in the abdominal cavity are abdominal surgeries (70 to 85% are attributed to previous operations). Inflammatory processes in the abdominal cavity can also result in adhesions

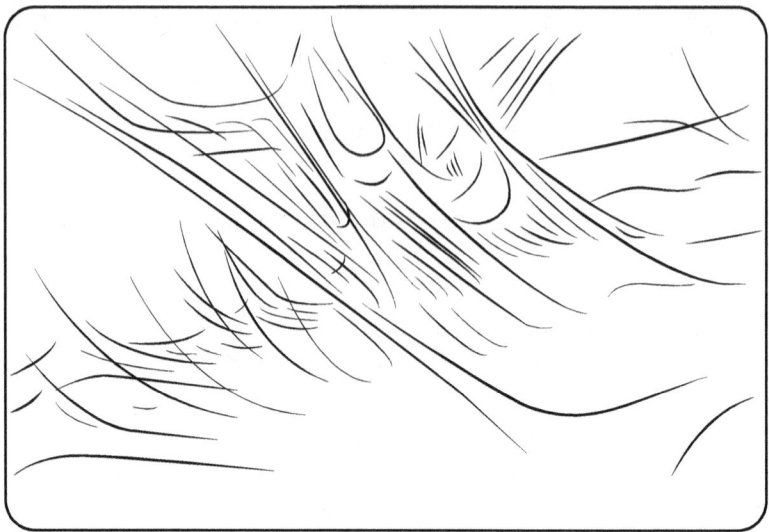

Fig. 1.3 Adhesions—flat structure

(Weibel and Majno 1973). During surgery, the body's inflammatory processes are influenced and changed in such a way that the adhesion processes necessary for the healing process or wound closure are specifically increased. At the same time, the body's own processes for breaking down excessive adhesions are reduced. The result can be different manifestations: from fine, flat adhesions (Fig. 1.3) to coarse, firm, band-like, cord-like (Ghahiry et al. 2012) adhesions of tissue layers of the abdominal cavity as well as between organs (Van Baal et al. 2016; Coccolini et al. 2013). In existing adhesions, both blood vessels and nerve fibers were found (Struller et al. 2017). Pronounced adhesions require a surgical cut with the scalpel to separate the adhered layers from each other. The result is a new wound of the mucous membrane with again the risk of triggering new adhesions and adhesions (Lindig 1922).

1.2.2 Structure of the Body Layers

To better understand how many tissue layers are affected during wound healing, I would like to first discuss their basic building block, the connective tissue, the structure and the most important subdivisions in our body. Adhesions can form between all these layers from the surface to the depth after an injury.

1.2.2.1 Connective Tissue

Connective tissue gives the body its shape. Layers of connective tissue, also called fascia, represent a chaotically dynamic network on a macroscopic to microscopic level, consisting of three-dimensional, fluid-filled mini-bubbles (medically: microvacuoles) and mini-fibers (medically: microfibrils) (Guimberteau and Armstrong 2016). This network is found as a basic framework throughout the body in denser and looser, flexible accumulations and connects all structures with each other. It also provides a large prepared repair kit to optimally support wound healing processes when needed. The network is also capable of transmitting forces, expanding and elongating, and then returning to its original state (Roman et al. 2013; Schleip et al. 2014). This mechanical property is determined by the tissue components collagen and elastin, which are developed and pronounced differently depending on the stress exerted on the connective tissue in the affected body region. Collagens have low elasticity and high tear resistance. They stabilize the connective tissue. Elastin, on the other hand, has the ability to extend up to 100 to 150% of the original length (about 20 to 30 times stronger than collagen) and then return to the original state (Pischinger 2010).

Pressure that arises in the layers of connective tissue is in turn absorbed by the mini-bubbles. They are arranged in different directions on several levels and reinforce the surrounding collagen framework. This allows good shock absorption and at the same time stabilizes the system. Accordingly, in tissue areas where a lot of pressure, force or movement must be managed, there are more smaller microvacuoles that distribute the acting forces harmoniously. This is intended to prevent overpressure in the mini-bubbles from resulting in fiber tears or permanent damage (Guimberteau 2014).

> **The Functionality of Connective Tissue**
>
> Without connective tissue, no connection and movement in the body would be possible. The versatile functionality of connective tissue is made possible by the following properties: It connects the body from head to foot and outside with inside. In the form of loose connective tissue, it supports the position of organs and at the same time allows their mobility due to its high sliding properties and capabilities by forming and ensuring sliding surfaces and spaces in the tissue. Movement is necessary to maintain the suppleness of the connective tissue and thus the health of the body.

As dense connective tissue, it solidifies into superficial and deep fascial layers, but also into ligaments or tendons up to cartilage and bones. Thus, connective tissue manages to generate flexibility and stability and thus enable mechanical interactions in the body between muscles, joints and organs etc. On the other hand, it connects the body from head to foot and outside with inside. Depending on the location, requirements and the impact of mechanical forces, the fibers align and are accordingly adapted and changed in the body if necessary (Geiger et al. 2001; Guimberteau and Armstrong 2016). Microscopically fine tissue fibers (with a diameter of 10 to 25 nm) can join together to form fiber bundles, which can then reach a diameter of several millimeters. To maintain this mobility, it is necessary that the tissue is kept versatile and constantly in motion. This starts with proper breathing, which mobilizes the whole body through many movement chains and includes any kind of everyday movement and sport. Under poor conditions, however, ball-like accumulations or densifications can occur in the connective tissue, such as adhesions (Pischinger 2010). Triggers include restricted movement stimuli or immobilizing the whole body or individual parts of the body for a longer period of time. Tissue injuries, traumas or acute and chronic inflammations also contribute and lead to the formation of adhesions. These reduce the mechanical properties and the ability to shift the loose connective tissue partially or completely. The tissue resistance increases and thus the tension in the tissue and the surrounding structures (von Heymann and Stecco 2016; Liedler 2017). Through its own sensors in the connective tissue, these changed tension pulls are perceived and the tissue is reinforced, changed and adapted according to the new loads (Langevin et al. 2004). To compensate for these tensions, the body develops special compensation patterns, such as individual protective postures or changed muscle loads. In the long run, this can then lead to overloading in the sense of chronic pain conditions.

1.2.2.2 The Skin

The skin is the largest organ of the human body. With an area of about two square meters, it covers the entire body. The outermost layer of the skin acts as a protective barrier against environmental factors such as bacteria, viruses, UV rays, and chemical substances. In the underlying layer, we find nerve endings, sebaceous glands, hair cells, and tiny blood vessels. Also located here are sensors that report the effects of mechanical stimuli and pain to the body. Below this is a layer that acts as an energy store and insulation against heat loss through fat deposits in the skin.

Under normal circumstances, our skin has a fine checkerboard structure typical for it on the surface. This serves to distribute mechanical loads well and dynamically to prevent injuries. We can all see this structure with the naked eye. Depending on the load, it becomes more pronounced in some places in the form of wrinkles as we age.

The fine checkerboard pattern on our skin surface, which extends into the deeper layers, allows mechanical tensions and forces to be absorbed and distributed in such a way that no damage occurs or the skin does not tear (Guimberteau and Armstrong 2016). If injuries to the skin do occur, complex local and systemic mechanisms cause rapid repair, even if the original mechanical characteristics cannot be fully restored and deviating scar patterns occur (Bordoni et al. 2023).

1.2.2.3 Fascia

1.2.2.3.1 Superficial Fascial Layer

The skin consists roughly of three layers, which merge fluidly with an underlying envelope layer of loose connective tissue and a fat layer—the superficial fascial layer. Several layers of fibers with different properties ensure stretching, elastic rebound, and mobility of the skin in relation to the musculoskeletal system. Due to the various fibers, tissue displacements and fiber stretches can happen complexly and multidimensionally at the same time (Abu-Hijleh et al. 2014).

The superficial fascia fulfills several functions. Due to its composition of fibers and subcutaneous fat tissue, it can absorb, intercept, and transmit applied pressure and displacement forces. In addition, surrounding subcutaneous fat serves as insulation against heat loss and as an energy store. Nerves and blood vessels are loosely and protected embedded between the sliding layers to ensure good supply and care of the tissue (Fede et al. 2018; Willard 2014a). Furthermore, the presence of a special fascia "kit" in the tissue ensures that in the event of an injury, the wound area is quickly and optimally supplied so that the wound is closed and adequate wound healing can take place (Correa-Gallegos et al. 2019).

1.2.2.3.2 Deep Fascial Layer

Deeper in the tissue, one finds a densification of the connective tissue. This is designed to transmit muscle tensions and movements or to be able to maintain this state. This layer is referred to as the deep fascial layer. To enable a corresponding fine-tuning in the dynamic movement apparatus between joints, muscles, bones, and the brain, the deep fascial layer is equipped with many different information receptors that provide feedback on the current stimulus load. These include sensors that provide precise information about mechanical loads and positions in space. These ensure that the tissue is always optimally adapted and that movements can take place smoothly and with minimal friction. On the other hand, this tissue is equipped with a high number of free nerve endings responsible for pain perception and report damaging influences, such as overloading, overstretching, inflammation, or injury, to the brain (Pavan et al. 2014; Schilder et al. 2014; Tesarz et al. 2011). In addition, special repair sets for scar formation in the fascial structures are also found here, which are specifically designed to ensure optimal wound healing (Correa-Gallegos et al. 2019; Schleip et al. 2014). Special cells in this fascial layer ensure a good balance in the tissue by creating good conditions for tissue build-up and breakdown and thus play an important role in wound healing processes. Other cells ensure the smoothness and frictionless shifting of the tissue layers by producing the lubricant hyaluron (Stecco et al. 2018). Overall, a large number of cells and components of the fascia work together complementarily and promotively exactly where movement must be able to take place. Specifically, this means: displacement forces, sliding movements, and pressure or tensile loads must be well balanced and transmitted to guarantee relaxed and complex power transmission and thus pain-free movement sequences (Schleip et al. 2014; Stecco et al. 2009).

1.2.2.3.3 The Functions of Fasciae

Fasciae cover important areas of responsibility in the body on several levels. They form a body-encompassing network that connects people from head to toe and from inside to outside. Through their movable properties, they offer protection against injury by ensuring that external influences such as pressure and tensile stress as well as shear forces can be well absorbed and redistributed.

The main task of the dense, deep fascia is the transmission and distribution of movements and muscle forces or the stabilization and anchoring of the large organs in the chest, abdomen, and pelvis. The deep fascial layer also serves as a guide and support layer for blood supply and lymphatic drainage and coherent feedback of the nervous system. In addition, it guarantees the mobility and smoothness of the tissue layers both among each other and in relation to the surrounding muscles, tendons, joints, bones, or organs. Many muscles are directly connected to the deep fascia. Thus, fascial systems and muscle chains can work together specifically to transmit forces from one body segment to the next and to tension and tighten involved movement systems. To be able to perceive movements precisely and accurately, optimally support, control, and carry them out, the deep fascia is richly interspersed with different information sensors. These include pain receptors that warn the body of overuse, inflammation, or traumatic events (Pavan et al. 2014; Willard 2014a).

> **The Main Functions of the Fasciae and Deep, Firm Tissue Layers**
> - Mobility through the sliding and displacement of the tissue layers to each other
> - Transmission and distribution of movement and muscle forces
> - Optimal movement coordination through continuity of muscle chains and fascial systems via the attachment of muscles to fasciae
> - Perception of one's own body position in space through information sensors for joint mechanics and movement perception
> - Perception of overwhelming stimuli and warning through pain sensors
> - Anchoring of organs in the pelvis
> - Stability for nerve conduction, blood supply, and lymphatic drainage

1.2.3 The Fascial System

In order to move and control the body precisely, we need, apart from the musculature, a specific guidance system: the so-called fascial system. This system consists of connective tissue and has the ability to distribute forces that we activate for movements evenly and dynamically throughout the body. This also ensures that the mobility and function of the tissues and organs are kept healthy and flexible. Because a constant alternation between tension and relaxation is necessary for both the renewal of connective tissue and the production of sliding mechanisms to keep the body agile and supple (Van den Berg 2014a, b).

Our body is enveloped and connected by this fascial system through a three-dimensional variable mechanical network of connective tissue and fascia from its surface to its depth. In this process, movable fascial layers with different density, orientation and texture, adapted to the respective body region, can be distinguished. With the help of special cells that have a certain muscle component (medically: myofibroblasts), the individual layers are able to generate tension in the fascial system and co-determine muscle activity (Bordoni and Zanier 2014). Even the smallest muscle fibers are enveloped and limited inside by the finest connective tissue, which allows the most precise adjustments, control and movement coordination. On the outside, the muscle is then surrounded by a fiber system that connects as a mechanical unit with the tendons, which in turn form a mechanical unit with the adjacent body structures.

The main task of the fascial system is to transmit and coordinate both mechanical forces and movements as well as to absorb loads in the sense of shock absorption. Organs are also stabilized in their place by this. Each fascial layer, in turn, consists of several sliding layers with different characteristics and their own production of lubricant (e.g., hyaluron). This enables smoothness, flexibility, a complex interplay and optimal transmission of forces.

This dynamic, harmonious interplay is also necessary to control inflammation and enable an optimal course of wound healing processes. The connective tissue is equipped with a wealth of information sensors that can recognize different stimuli, such as pressure, vibration and pain. This allows the fascial system to recognize both mechanical and potentially harmful stimuli and tissue changes, such as those that occur in adhesions and scarring, and, if necessary, to convert and transmit them into pain information.

Incorrect or premature strain on tissue structures after injuries can negatively affect the wound healing process. "Wrong" impulses can overwhelm the tissue and thus lead to the activation of pain processes. A deficient or useless tissue remodeling due to unfavorable scar formation or chronic inflammatory processes can overload the fascial system and thus cause chronic pain conditions (Van den Berg 2014b; Bordoni and Zanier 2014). Movement = Health Flexible, supple, movable, adaptable connective tissue is essential for our health, relaxed and frictionless movements in the body and freedom from pain.

1.3 Sliding Mechanisms in the Body—Mobility of Connective Tissue

Loose connective tissue can be found everywhere in the body where sliding properties of tissue are needed for movement. Here, different special sliding systems allow almost frictionless sliding of muscles and tendons.

> **Example of Mobility and Sliding of Tissue**
> Take your wrist, for example. All the movements you can make there are controlled by muscles and tendons in the forearm. These must shorten and tense there so that you can move your wrist. If you now bend or stretch the wrist or tilt it sideways, you will not notice any displacement of the skin or tendons on the forearm despite the muscle shortening. Any tissue displacements happen invisibly under the skin due to the tissue's ability to slide and move unnoticed relative to each other.

Skin, tendons, fascia, and muscles are connected by loose connective tissue, which at the same time always allows movement. As a result, tendons can move several centimeters between tissue structures without this movement becoming visible on the skin (Guimberteau et al. 2010). Responsible for this is a system of mini-bubbles and tissue fibers that form delicate to firm connections as needed. Nerves, blood vessels, and lymph vessels are integrated into these structures in such a way that they can easily move along with movements. In this way, their continuity and a stable vascular supply in the tissue are guaranteed. Parallel to this, the mini-bubbles serve as shock absorbers, being able to withstand occurring pressure forces, compressions, stretches, and shear forces (Guimberteau et al. 2007).

The flexible tissue framework provides the stability, while a gel-like base substance in the tissue allows reshaping during movement. The sliding system operates in a functional, three-dimensional chaos, is interconnected in many ways, changes along force lines, expands and widens, and always returns to its original form. During movements, the shape of the network of fibers and mini-bubbles is continuously adapted to the need, allowing this network to constantly reform and adapt to the respective physical conditions (Guimberteau and Armstrong 2016; Guimberteau 2014).

> **Moving and Sliding in Tissue**
> - Means three-dimensional maximally flexible tissue connections in all directions and with all surrounding structures (like a three-dimensional spider web)
> - Means extending the tissue fibers and then returning to the original form
> - Means that fibers can connect and extend with other fibers, to separate after the load and return to the original form
> - Means, the more movement is needed in a body area, the more lubricant like hyaluron is produced there

As an elemental component of loose connective tissue, the lubricant hyaluron significantly contributes to the maintenance of sliding layers. High proportions of hyaluron were measured in areas where a lot of movement and suppleness is needed, such as around our joints (Fede et al. 2018; McCombe et al. 2001). An increased hyaluron concentration can—depending on additional factors such as existing movement, shear or pressure impulses—contribute to an improvement of the sliding layers. Lack of movement has the opposite effect: Immobilization or too little movement (traumatic or inflammatory) can lead to changes in the hyaluron concentration. This densification of hyaluron increases the tissue's readiness to create adhesions (Cowman et al. 2015), which then make sliding difficult or even prevent it.

To summarize: In general, the special structure of loose connective tissue allows mobility within the fascial system, thereby enabling sliding ability and flexibility. At the same time, the tissue can absorb pressure, while deep fascial layers generate stability in the tissue. The entire connective tissue continuously ensures the best possible balance between flexibility and stability.

1.4 Wound Healing

For the wound healing, the body needs certain inflammatory processes. What does this mean? Upon closer inspection, these inflammations are defined processes that remodel, repair, renew, and restore the tissue, with the aim of restoring the original functional state as best as possible. They always start with an acute inflammation phase, after which new tissue is built up in the affected area. This complex remodeling process is crucial for the wound or tissue healing of small and large injuries, for bruises, for muscle building, and other regeneration processes in the body. After an injury, the body or the affected area is continuously adapted and changed to the individual needs over a period of about one year. In short: Without inflammation, there is no effective repair, no remodeling, and no desired reconstruction. Nowadays, inflammation is often very negatively connoted in our minds. It is overlooked that complication-free inflammations are fundamentally a completely normal and important part of the renewal processes in the body. Inflammatory process = Healing process = Remodeling process Without inflammation, the body does not initiate wound healing processes and tissue remodeling.

So, the "bruises" known to all of us also mean a wound in the tissue that triggers tissue renewal. And muscle soreness is, in the true sense, a tissue remodeling of our body.

1.4.1 Physiological or "Normal" Wound Healing (See Fig. 1.4)

1.4.1.1 Skin Wound Healing

The wound healing of the skin depends on different factors. A visible scar forms when both the skin and the deeper layers of skin are affected by the injury. How long the healing phase lasts or the size of the scars that form is usually based on the size and depth of the wound or surgical incision,

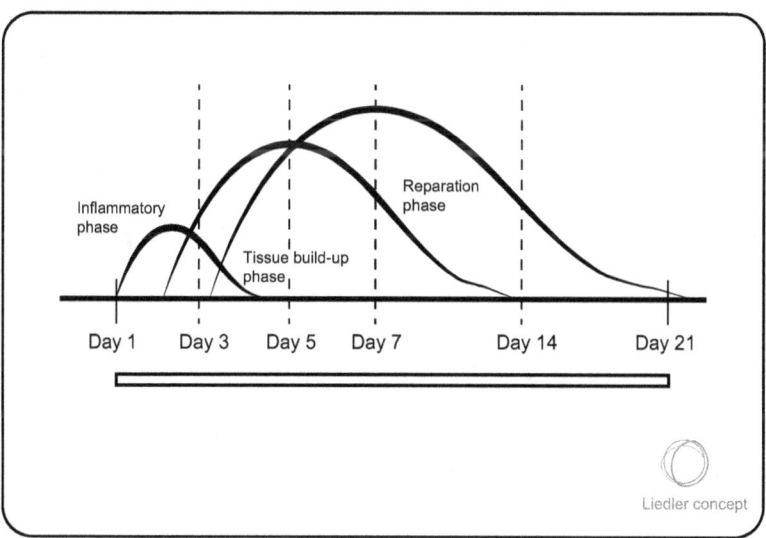

Fig. 1.4 Phases of wound healing. (© 2022 Liedler-Konzept)

or on occurring infections. Accordingly, the treatment forms are different. Without complications, this wound usually heals within six to 14 days. The final strength of the tissue is only established after a few more weeks and months. While a superficial wound is primarily closed by the deposition of new tissue, the formation of tissue components in deep wounds is taken over by fasciae. With the help of prefabricated "repair kits" made of the required cell types, scar formation is significantly enabled and supported by the affected tissue and the fasciae.

In general, wound healing is described in three overlapping phases with a duration of 14 days, with the peak of inflammation or remodeling occurring between the third and fifth day. The healing of a skin wound happens from the outer wound edges inward. This means that the larger the skin wound, the longer the path until the wound is well closed and healed.

1.4.1.1.1 Inflammatory Phase

Every wound healing begins with an acute inflammation. Without an inflammatory process, there is no healing. In the first phase (day one to five), it ensures that the bleeding is stopped, the wound is cleaned, the destroyed tissue is glued together for reconstruction, and a good supply of the tissue is guaranteed. The first adhesions occur in the healing process within the first three hours. They are supposed to interweave the adjacent tissue surfaces with each other and repair the damage. The wound is stabilized and a crust forms on the outside. Within 24 h, a temporary replacement tissue surface is formed. This acute phase of remodeling is often accompanied by redness and overheating of the injured tissue. The accompanying swelling irritates nerve endings in the tissue, triggers pain, and restricts movement in the affected area. As a result, protective postures often occur so that the tissue damage can be well, efficiently, and quickly processed in the first phase of healing (Asmussen and Söllner 2010).

1.4.1.1.2 Tissue Building Phase

Subsequently (day five to 21), the body focuses on the formation of new tissue and blood vessels. Special cells, which have the ability to contract, move the injured tissue areas towards each other, stabilize them, and simultaneously form new tissue (Van den Berg 2014b). The tissue regeneration reaches its peak after six to 16 days and continues for several more weeks. The goal is to restore the optimal strength of the tissue (Asmussen and

Söllner 2010). In this phase, the initial signs of inflammation already subside and the increasing mobility supports the restoration of functionality and flexibility in the tissue.

1.4.1.1.3 Repair Phase

The final phase of wound healing lasts up to a year. Its goal is to further adapt the connective tissue to the stresses and remodel it accordingly (Van den Berg 2014b). Once the skin repair is fully completed, the crust dissolves and all excess cells in the scar are broken down, making it appear whitish in the process (Wight and Potter-Perigo 2011).

> **Chronic pain that occurs a year after surgery can very well still be related to the surgery**
> Interestingly, as a therapist, I often observe in practice that pain symptoms and tensions related to surgeries often only become disturbingly noticeable after about a year. So just at the time when the repair processes are completed. At this point, however, few affected people and doctors attribute occurring chronic pain conditions to previous surgeries.

1.4.1.2 Wound Healing of the Abdominal Membrane Sac

The abdominal membrane is lined with mucous membrane. What does this mean for wound healing? The healing of the mucous membrane in the abdominal cavity is similar to that of the skin, but it is completed within five to ten days regardless of the wound size. This is mainly due to the fact that new tissue is formed simultaneously everywhere, that is, both at the edge of the wound and in its center (DiZerega 2000).

During the healing process, the injured tissue layers are glued together to subsequently form new tissue and new blood vessels. Adequate oxygen supply to the cells is crucial for good tissue restoration. In the abdominal cavity, islands of new tissue that are firmly connected to each other can already be seen from day 2. From the fourth day, this network is already consolidated. Normally, the initial support structures and adhesions are dissolved again through targeted degradation processes. By day 10, the wound is healed regardless of its size and the process is largely completed.

What aspects are relevant here in the abdominal cavity? Organs should be able to move with as little friction as possible in the abdominal cavity. Therefore, it is functionally important that their mucous surface does not stick or connect with adjacent tissue layers. A wound closure in the abdominal cavity is therefore successful when a stable cell layer has been formed that can slide and is free and easily movable in relation to the organs inside the abdominal membrane sac (DiZerega 2000).

1.4.2 Pathophysiological or Adverse Wound Healing

Wound healing does not always proceed optimally. Pathophysiological wound healing is referred to when the healing is delayed due to complications and the affected area cannot be functionally restored accordingly. What does this mean for the body layers we are considering?

1.4.2.1 Pathophysiological or Adverse Skin Wound Healing

The healing of skin wounds can be delayed by infections or other complications if they interfere with wound closure due to excessive tissue loss or high tensions in the area of the wound. Also, shredded wound edges, purulence, foreign bodies in the wound, or the reinfection of an already closed wound can massively impair wound closure. In any case, an *"extensive, retracted, cosmetically unsatisfactory, and functionally, especially at the joints, disturbing scar."* arises (Asmussen and Söllner 2010, p. 58). In the course of wound healing processes, the wound surface is filled with repair tissue and converted into scar tissue, which is impairing as the scar tissue is always formed the same, regardless of whether skin, muscles, or tendons are repaired (Guimberteau and Armstrong 2016) and the tissue strength can only be restored to a maximum of 80%. The chaotic, thickened, and functionally unsuitable arrangement of new tissue additionally reduces elasticity, flexibility, and suppleness. Different qualities of scars are the result (Asmussen and Söllner 2010).

Under normal circumstances, the skin has a fine checkerboard structure typical for it. As already described above, it serves to distribute mechanical loads well and dynamically to prevent injury.

If there is a change in this fine structure during wound healing in the sense of thickened, broad fibers due to scars, adhesions, or proliferations, this leads to a lack of mobility in the superficial, deep, and adjacent tissue. The supply of the tissue is impaired and suppleness is lost. This is perceived as a pulling or tingling sensation. Due to the adverse compactions of the tissue, subtle inflammations also persist. These often manifest themselves through itching of the scar and create further tensions in the tissue. It becomes complicated for the body to satisfactorily complete the healing process (Guimberteau and Armstrong 2016).

> **Recognizing Adverse Wound Healing**
> - Delayed wound healing
>   In case of high tissue loss, shredded wound edges, purulence, foreign bodies, reinfection of already closed wounds
>   – TIP: Disinfect and consult a doctor
> - Delayed wound closure
>   Often due to the formation of bruises and accumulation of fluid, which MECHANICALLY push apart the wound edges
>   – TIP: Careful handling of the body and the scar in the first weeks
> - Excessive scars
>   Formation due to strong tensile forces acting on the young tissue
>   – TIP: after the operation: silicone patches, compression bandages, mindful movements, avoidance of strong muscular strains until the surgeon gives the all-clear for sports
> - Keloid
>   Complex disturbance of tissue remodeling due to persistent inflammation and high pain sensitivity
>   – TIP: always consult a doctor, closely monitor stress levels—many factors are always involved

1.4.2.2 Pathophysiological or Adverse Healing of the Abdominal Membrane Sac

Adhesions in the abdominal cavity often occur after surgeries or inflammations of the abdominal cavity (Arung et al. 2011).

In this case, as a result of a wound, the firm cell connection of the surface of the mucosal tissue detaches from the underlying membrane and forms open, sticky surfaces. These can connect with adjacent tissue surfaces and organs to form dense adhesions. This process is intensified during surgeries, especially when there is bleeding (DiZerega 2000). This disrupts normal wound healing and tissue remodeling. During the healing process, it may happen that initial adhesions are not immediately dissolved, but remain and become solidified. New tissue tracts are formed in the abdominal cavity, which either serve as thin connective tissue layers or as firm, dense tissue strands with blood vessels and nerve strands, or as adhesions connecting two organs. These are the adhesions in the abdominal cavity (medically: peritoneal adhesions) already described above (Coccolini et al. 2013).

References

Abu-Hijleh, Marwan, A. S. Dharap, P. F. Harris. 2014. „Fascia superficialis". *Lehrbuch Faszien*, herausgegeben von R. Schleip, T. W. Findley, L. Chaltow, P. A. Huijing, 1. Auflage, 15–18. München: Elsevier GmbH.

Arung, Willy, Michel Meurisse, Olivier Detry. 2011. „Pathophysiology and prevention of postoperative peritoneal adhesions". *World Journal of Gastroenterology* 17 (41): 4.545–53.

Asmussen, Peter D., Brigitte Söllner. 2010. Die Prinzipien der Wundheilung. Bd. Sonderausgabe. Embrach: Kammerlander.

Bordoni, Bruno, Emiliano Zanier. 2014. „Clinical and symptomatological reflections: The fascial system." Journal of Multidisciplinary Healthcare, Nr. 7: 401–411.

Bordoni, Bruno, Escher A.R., Girgenti G.T., Tobbi F., Bonanzinga R. Osteopathic Approach for Keloids and Hypertrophic Scars. Cureus. 2023 Sep 7;15(9):e44815. https://doi.org/10.7759/cureus.44815. PMID: 37692181; PMCID: PMC10483258.

Bouffard, N. A., K. Cutroneo, G. J. Badger et al. 2008. „Tissue Stretch Decreases Soluble TGF-β1 and Type-1 Procollagen in Mouse Subcutaneous Connective Tissue: Evidence From Ex Vivo and In Vivo Models". *J Cell Physiol* 214 (2): 389–95.

Carano, A., G. Siciliani. 1996. „Effects of continuous and intermittend forces on human fibroblasts in vitro". Eur J Orthod 18 (1): 19–26.

Cheong, Y. C., S. M. Laird, J. B. Shelton et al. 2001. „Peritoneal healing and adhesion formation/reformation". *Human Reproduction Update* 7 (6): 556–66.

Coccolini, Frederico, Luca Ansaloni, Roberto Manfredi et al. 2013. „Peritoneal adhesion index (PAI): proposal of a score for the ‚ignored iceberg' of medicine and surgery". *World Journal of Emergency Surgery*, Nr. 8: 1–6.

Correa-Gallegos, D., D. Jiang, S. Christ, P. Ramesh, H. Ye, J. Wannemacher, S.K. Gopal, et al. 2019. „Patch repair of deep wounds by mobilized fascia". *Nature*. https://doi.org/10.1038/s41586-019-1794-y.

Cowman, M. K., T. A. Schmidt, P. Raghavan, A. Stecco. 2015. „Viscoelastic Properties of Hyaluronan in Physiological Conditions". *F1000Research* 4 (655). https://doi.org/10.12688/f1000research.6885.1.

DiZerega, Gere S. 2000. *Peritoneum, peritoneal healing, and adhesion formation. Peritoneal surgery*. Bd. Peritoneal surgery. New York: Springer-Verlag. 3–37.

DiZerega, G.S. & Campeau, J. D. (2001). Peritoneal repair and post-surgical adhesion formation. Human Reproduction Update, 7, 547–55.

Fede, C., A. Angelini, R. Stern, V. Macchi et al. 2018. „Quantification of hyaluronan in human fasciae: variations with function and anatomical site". *Journal of Anatomy* 233 (4): 552–56. https://doi.org/10.1111/joa.12866.

Fourie, W. J. 2014. „Operationen und Narbenbildung". *Lehrbuch Faszien*, herausgegeben von R. Schleip, T. W. Findely, L. Chaitow, P. A. Huijing, 1. Auflage, 308–15. München: Elsevier GmbH.

Geiger, Benjamin, Alexander Bershadsky, Roumen Pankov, Kenneth M. Yamada. 2001. „Transmembrane Crosstalk Between the Extracellular Matrix-Cytoskeleton Crosstalk". *Nature Reviews Molechular Cell Biology* 2: 793–805.

Ghahiry, Ata, Farimah Rezaei, Reza Karimi Khouzani, Mansoor Ashrafinia. 2012. „Comparative analysis of long-term outcomes of Misgav-Ladach technique cesarean section and traditional cesarean section". *The Journal of Obstetrics and Gynaecology Research* 38 (10): 1.235–39.

Guimberteau, J. C. 2014. „Das subkutane und epitendinöse Gewebe des multimikrovakuolären Gleitsystems". *Lehrbuch Faszien*, herausgegeben von R. Schleip, T. W. Findely, L. Chaitow, P. A. Huijing, 1. Auflage, 106–8. München: Urban & Fischer.

Guimberteau, J. C., J. P. Delage, D. A. Mcgrouther, J. K. F. Wong. 2010. „The microvacuolar system: how connective tissue sliding works". The Journal of Hand Surgery, 2010, 35. Auflage, Abschn. 8.

———, Colin Armstrong. 2016. *Faszien Architektur des menschlichen Fasziengewebes*. 1. Auflage, Berlin: KVM – Der Medizinverlag.

Guimberteau, J. C., J. Bakhach, B. Panconi, S. Rouzaud. 2007. „A fresh look at vascularized flexor tendon transfers: concept, technical aspects and results". *J Plast Reconstructr Aesthet Surg* 60 (7): 793–810.

———, J. P. Delage, D. A. Mcgrouther, J. K. F. Wong. 2010. „The microvacuolar system: how connective tissue sliding works". *The Journal of Hand Surgery*, 2010, 35. Auflage, Abschn. 8.

Helsmoortel, Jerome, Thomas Hirth, Peter Wührl. 2002. Lehrbuch der viszeralen Osteopathie Peritoneale Organe. Stuttgart: Georg Thieme Verlag.

Heymann, Wolfgang von, Carla Stecco. 2016. „Fasziale Dysfunktionen". *Manuelle Medizin* 54: 303–6. https://doi.org/10.1007/s00337-016-0172-1.

Ingber, Donald E. 2008a. „Tensegrity and mechanotransduction". *Journal of Bodywork & Movement Therapies* 12: 198–200.

Langevin, H.M., C. Cornbrooks, D. J. Taatjes. 2004. „Fibroblast form a body-wide cellular network". Histochem Cell Biol 122: 7–15.

Liedler, Michaela 2017. „Einfluss von postoperativen Adhäsionen nach Sektio auf chronischen Low Back Pain – eine Pilotstudie". Masterthese, Krems: DUK.

———. 2020. *„Peritoneale Adhäsionen – Fasziale Behandlung nach dem Liedler-Konzept"*. Berlin, Heidelberg: Springer Verlag GmbH.

Lindig, Paul. 1922. „Über die Entstehung, Bedeutung und Behandlung von Adhäsionen im Beckenbauchraum". Klinische Wochenzeitschrift 1 (22): 421–23.

McCombe, D., T. Brown, J. Slavin, W.A. Morrison. 2001. „The Histochemical Structure Of The Deep Fascia And Its Structural Response To Surgery". Journal of Hand Surgery 26B (2): 89–97.

Pados, G., C. A. Venetis, K. Almaloglou, B. C. Tarlatzis. 2010. „Prevention of intra-peritoneal adhesions in gynaecological surgery: theory and evidence". Reproductive BioMedicine Online, Nr. 21: 290–303. https://doi.org/10.1016/j.rbmo.2010.04.021.

Pavan, G. Piero, Antonio Stecco, Robert Stern, Carla Stecco. 2014. „Painful Connections: Densification Versus Fibrosis of Fascia". Curr Pain Headache Rep 18 (441): 1–8.

Pischinger, Alfred. 2010. Das System der Grundregulation. Neu herausgegeben von Hartmut Heine. 12. Auflage, Stuttgart: Karl F. Haug Verlag.

Roman, Max, Hans Chaudhry, Bruce Bukiet, Antonio Stecco et al. 2013. „Mathematical Analysis of the Flow of Hyaluronic Acid around Fascia During Manual Therapy Motions". The Journal of the American Osteopathic Association 113 (8): 600–10.

Schilder, A., U. Hoheisel, W. Magerl, J. Benrath, et al. 2014. „Sensory findings after stimulation of the thoracolumbar fascia with hypertonic saline suggest its contribution to low back pain". Pain 155: 222–31.

Schleip, R. 2003a. „Fascial plasticity – a new neurobiological explanation, Part 1". Journal of Bodywork & Movement Therapies 7 (1): 11–19.

Schleip, R. 2003b. „Fascial plasticity – a new neurobiological explanation, Part 2". Journal of Bodywork & Movement Therapies 7 (2): 104–16.

Schleip, R., T. W Findley, L. Chaltow (Hrsg.). 2014. „Lehrbuch Faszien". 1. Auflage, München: Elsevier GmbH.

———, H. Jäger, W. Klingler. 2014. „Die Faszie lebt: wie Faszientonus und -struktur von Zellen moduliert werden". Lehrbuch Faszien, herausgegeben von R. Schleip, T. W. Findely, L. Chaitow, P. A. Huijing, 1. Auflage, 115–20. München: Elsevier GmbH.

Standley, Paul R., Kate R. Meltzer. 2008. „In vitro modeling of repetive motion strain and manual medicine treatments: Potential roles for pro- and anti-inflammatory cytocines". Journal of Bodywork & Movement Therapies 12: 201–3.

Stecco, Carla, C. Fede, V. Macchi, A. Porzionato, et al. 2018. „The Fasciacytes: A New Cell Devoted to Fascial Gliding Regulation". Clinical Anatomy. https://doi.org/10.1002/ca.23072.

Stecco, A., A. Meneghini, R. Stern, C. Stecco. 2014. „Ultrasonography in myofascial neck pain: randomized clinical trial for diagnosis and follow-up". Surg Radiol Anat 36: 243–53.

———, Piero G. Pavan, Andrea Porzionato, Veronica Macchi et al. 2009. „Mechanics of crural fascia: from anatomy to sonstitutive modelling". Surg Radiol Anat 31: 523–29. https://doi.org/10.1007/s00276-009-0474-2.

Stöckl, Diana. 2019. „Osteopathische Aspekte von Interozeption und Emotion". DO – Deutsche Zeitschrift für Osteopathie 17 (02): 25-31.

Struller, F., F.-J. Weinreich, P. Horvath, M.-K. Kokkalis, S. Beckert et al. 2017. „Peritoneal innervation: embryology and functional anatomy". Pleura Peritoneum 2 (4): 153–61.

Tesarz, J., U. Hoheisel, B. Wiedenhofer, S. Mense. 2011. „SENSORY INNERVATION OF THE THORACOLUMBAR FASCIA IN RATS AND HUMANS". Neuroscience 194: 302–8.
Threlkeld, A. Joseph. 1992. „The Effects of Manual Therapy on Connective Tissue". Journal of the American Physical Therapy Association, Nr. 72: 893–902.
Tozzi, Paolo, D. Bongiorno, C. Vitturini. 2011. „Fascial release effects on patients with non-specific cervical or lumbar pain". Journal of Bodywork & Movement Therapies 15 (4): 405–16.
Trindade, V. L., P. A. Martins, S. Santos, M. P. Parente et al. 2012. „Experimental study of the influence of senescence in the biomechanical properties of the temporal tendon and deep temporal fascia based on uniaxial tension tests". Journal of Biomechanics 45: 199–201.
Van Baal, J. O. A. M., K. K. Van de Vijver, R. Niewland, C. J. F. Van Noorden, et al. 2016. „The histophysiology and pathophysiology of the peritoneum". Tissue and Cell 49: 95–105.
Van den Berg, F. 2014a. „Die Extrazellulärmatrix". Lehrbuch Faszien, herausgegeben von R. Schleip, T. W. Findely, L. Chaitow, P. A. Huijing, 1. Auflage, 121–25. München: Elsevier GmbH.
Van den Berg, F. 2014b. „Die Physiologie der Faszie". Lehrbuch Faszien, herausgegeben von R. Schleip, T. W. Findely, L. Chaitow, P. A. Huijing, 1. Auflage, 110–14. München: Elsevier GmbH.
Weibel, M.-A., G. Majno. 1973. „Peritoneal adhesions and their relation to abdominal surgery: A postmortem study". American Journal of Surgery 126 (3): 345–53.
Wight, Thomas N., Susan Potter-Perigo. 2011. „The extracellular matrix: an active or passive player in fibrosis?" American Journal of Physiology – Gastrointestinal Liver Physiology 301 (6): G950–55.
Willard, F. H. 2014a. „Die somatische Faszie". Lehrbuch Faszien, herausgegeben von R. Schleip, T. W. Findely, L. Chaitow, P. A. Huijing, 1. Auflage, 9–14. München: Elsevier GmbH.
Willard, F. H. 2014b. „Die viszerale Faszie". Lehrbuch Faszien, herausgegeben von R. Schleip, T. W. Findely, L. Chaitow, P. A. Huijing, 1. Auflage, 39–41. München: Elsevier GmbH.

2

Consequences of Surgeries

2.1 Why do Adhesions Occur Particularly during Surgeries?

As is now clearly proven, adhesions in the abdominal cavity occur with a frequency of 50 to 95%. Different and complex mechanisms ensure that adhesions form during a surgery.

1. A major factor is the injury to the originally smooth cell layer on the mucous membranes of the abdominal cavity. If it is injured, the connective tissue develops a strong tendency to adhere to the adjacent tissue layers and organs during wound healing.

Although there have been and continue to be many attempts by both science and practical medicine to prevent these adhesions, no suitable method has been found to date.

2. The larger the operation, the more excessive are the inflammatory reactions with which the body responds to this internal injury. As a result of these inflammatory mechanisms, the risk of adhesion also increases. Blood in the surgical field also promotes the formation of adhesions and attachments.
3. How should we imagine this? Simply put, the body initiates an almost excessive healing process: At the beginning, the wound is chaotically

adhered during wound healing to effect a rapid wound closure. Overall, there is an increased formation of new tissue. Once the wound is closed, the excess tissue connections, i.e., adhesions, are normally broken down. However, this process is disrupted during operations, which consequently leads to excessive adhesions remaining in the tissue and being converted and consolidated into attachments between fascial tissue guide layers and/or the sliding layers of the abdominal cavity or organs. Over time, these are then organized into a permanent tissue with sensitive nerve fibers and vessels. (DiZerega and Campeau 2001; Pados et al. 2010)

2.2 Small Skin Incision (Laparoscopy) versus Large Skin Incision (Laparotomy)

2.2.1 Laparoscopy—the small skin incision

Nowadays, large and small operations in the abdominal cavity or on joints are hidden under small skin incisions, which are performed using laparoscopy. Laparoscopic operations have the great advantage that they cause less destruction of skin and mucosal tissue (see Fig. 2.1). The smaller wounds

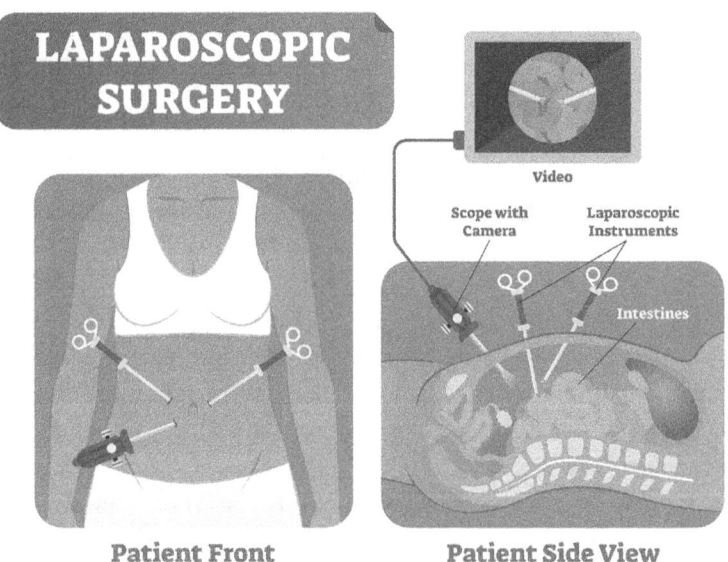

Fig. 2.1 Laparoscopy—the small skin incision. (© 2022 Liedler-Konzept/iStock: Getty Images)

can heal faster. However, it should be mentioned here that the abdominal cavity is filled with gas for the operation, which in turn can dry out the mucous membranes and provoke adhesions. Another danger associated with the "small operation" is that the actual size and wound of the surgical field is underestimated, as it is invisible in the depth of the body. Every wound inside is as large, wide, and complex as the surgical intervention requires to repair the respective damage. Despite the hardly noticeable small scar from the outside, complex and extensive adhesions can still occur inside the body.

Potential chronic pain conditions are then hardly associated with the "small operation". Typical statements are "I only had a small operation. It certainly has no influence and nothing to do with my symptoms".

2.2.2 Laparotomy—the large abdominal incision

In a laparotomy (see Fig. 2.2), a large skin incision is made, which unmistakably indicates the extent of the surgery. Compared to a laparoscopic procedure, it is not only more visible on the skin. Even inside the body, it can be associated with a stronger formation of adhesions. Depending on the size of the skin incision, the formation of the scar permanently leads to a deteriorated tissue situation in terms of mobility and suppleness on the skin surface. In addition, after a laparotomy, there is a strong tendency for

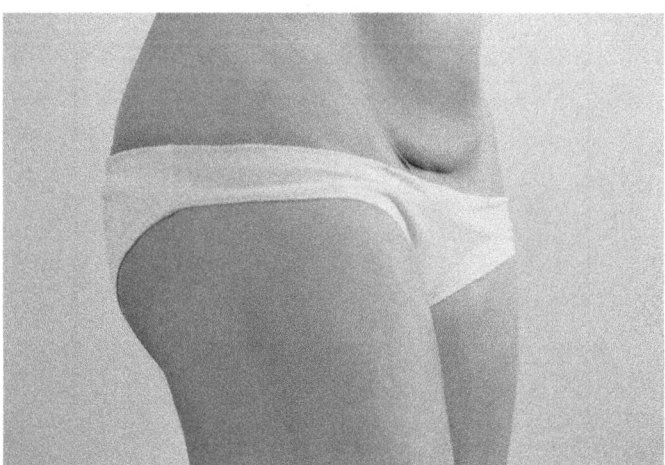

Fig. 2.2 Laparotomy—the large abdominal incision. (© 2021 Liedler-Konzept/ Photographer: Schaur)

concrete adhesion chains to form, which, starting from the skin and continuing over the superficial and deep tissue layers, form connections and adhesions deep into the abdominal cavity. The optical result is often a visible retraction of the scar into the depth and noticeable restrictions in the movement system.

2.3   Effects of Scars and Adhesions on the Body (see Fig. 2.3)

How do adhesions relate to tension in other parts of the body?
Adhesions can be imagined like a knot in a T-shirt. A normally loose fabric no longer falls loosely once it is knotted. Visible creases are created, which

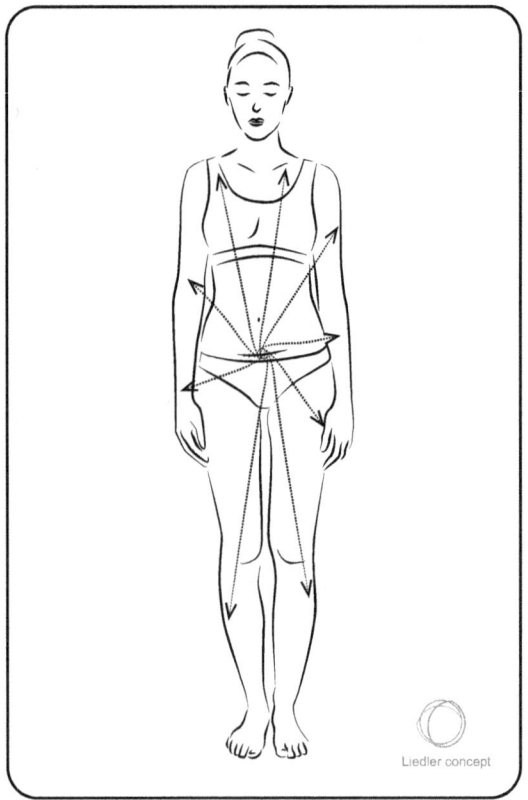

Fig. 2.3 Influence of adhesions on the body. (© 2023 Liedler-Konzept)

extend far beyond the knot and spread in all directions. This is how one can imagine the effects of adhesions pictorially: A knot in the body and the associated tensions that run from there in all directions. Anyone who tries it out with a fabric knot in the abdominal area will notice that the tension of the fabric extends up to the shoulders. If you have tucked the T-shirt into your pants, it may be that the fabric is pulled out of the pants again by the knot. This means that the entire fabric of the T-shirt reacts to the knot. Comparable tensile stresses occur in our body with adhesions in the connective tissue. But the body cannot open this knot again or simply take off the T-shirt. The tensions persist. The body must find a new balance. Individual movements are thereby restricted or unpleasantly changed. Tensions that can be felt correspond exactly to the places where chronic tension and pain conditions develop in the body over time.

Now imagine that there is not just one surgery in your life history, but that more knots are added: How comfortable or tight does your body feel now? How well and freely can you move now?

Surgical interventions, inflammations, injuries, swellings, traumas, chronic irritations and pain as well as immobilization, protective postures or aging cause changes in the sliding system of the connective tissue. While in normal cases fibers and mini bubbles react flexibly to changes in shape, intensive traumas, large wound fields, injuries or tissue overstretching can cause overload, which destroys the *"[...] precise interplay of the connective tissue structure. Bleeding, swelling, lymphatic effusion and excessive blood circulation disturb the mechanical balance, and increase the resistance in the tissue. Movements are difficult and require more strength. If tissue adhesions occur due to trauma or immobilization, mobility is further restricted. [...] The result is a permanent functional impairment."* (Guimberteau 2014, p. 107).

This negative influence on the connective tissue leads to persistent mechanical tensions, which always also cause a deterioration of the surrounding fascial tissue sliding layers and structures. What are the consequences then? The local tension is transferred to the involved fascia and muscle system and the body develops corresponding compensation mechanisms. As a result, symptoms may develop that occur far away from the triggering source.

Because a permanent tension in body areas, which per se are not designed to always be under increased load, can trigger the release of inflammation-promoting substances. Swellings occur in the tissue, which in turn generate further stiffness and tension in the tissue, which further restrict the sliding layers. This cycle irritates further pain receptors, eventually triggers pain and in the end and protective postures. Over time, complex and protracted chronic pain conditions can develop (Bordoni and Zanier 2014).

2.3.1 Effects of Scars on the Body

Scars always represent a visible change in the skin surface. In the best case, only recognizable as a thin, white, movable line, the scar can present itself differently. It can be uniformly said that scar tissue, as unorganized filler tissue, is always produced in the same way, regardless of whether skin, muscle or tendons are affected.

> **Identifying Irritated Scars**
> - ReddenedScar
> - Itchy, flaky, bulging scar
> - Thickenings, hardenings, lumps under the skin
> - Retraction of the scar
> - Hard scar strand
> - Formation of a "overhanging tissue fold" over the scar
> - Hypersensitivity of the scar or pain
> - Numbness of the scar
> - Pressure sensitivity of the scar (clothing presses uncomfortably)
> - Weather sensitivity
> - Feeling of being cut off
> - Pulling sensation in the scar area at rest or in motion
> - Formation of a shiny red Keloid scar (= excessive formation of scar tissue)

Due to disordered, thickened collagen fibers, scar tissue always loses elasticity and flexibility (Asmussen and Söllner 2010). The "optimal" scar is soft, white, and movable, can be touched without agitation, and integrates inconspicuously into the surrounding body system.

Unfortunately, however, scars can become noticeable in optical, mechanical, or sensitive ways. Instinctively, the affected person feels that something with the scar is not as it should be. An irritated scar can draw attention to itself through redness, thickening, hardening, retraction, and/or the formation of a "overhanging tissue fold" or also through changes in sensitivity and pain. Redness always indicates the lack of completion of repair processes in the tissue. Even if no pain is associated with it, redness can be associated with ongoing inflammatory processes and increased blood flow. The remodeling processes during scar formation can lead to a continuous collagen secretion, which is often palpable as a hard scar strand or hardening. Another consequence can be irritation of free nerve endings, which in turn maintain the cycle of irritation. What does this mean for the affected person? Newly activated pain sensors and nerve injuries caused by the skin incision can lead to permanent pressure sensitivity. There can also be increased sensitivity or even complete loss of sensitivity, i.e., numb insensitivity. A scar that flakes, itches, or is weather-sensitive also indicates that irritations and remodeling processes are still present in the affected area at a micro level.

Retractions and the "overhanging tissue fold" occur when the layers not only adhere to the surface but also to the underlying tissue layers. Since the tissue normally contracts during the healing process and the incision is not only on the surface but extends deep into the tissue, there is a compaction of these chained layers towards the depth of the tissue or abdominal cavity during the healing process. Visible from the outside on the body is then an indentation, like with a belt that is too tight. The loose tissue above the scar or the too tight belt appears optically like a thick "bulge". Often this bulge is coupled underneath with a hard scar strand and with noticeable lumps and hardenings in the depth of the scar tissue.

These less elastic adhesions of the tissue layers can in turn develop tension pulls that act on the young scar and promote the formation of raised, bulging scars.

In the worst case, this leads to the development of a so-called Keloid scar, in which persistent inflammations continuously cause scar growth and pain. Why keloid scars form is not yet fully understood. However, it is most likely due to a regulatory disorder of collagen metabolism (Bordoni et al. 2023).

Depending on the severity of the scar and also on how the affected person deals with their own, altered body area, the symptoms of scars can vary. They range from pain and an uncomfortable pulling sensation to unnoticed protective postures and compensation patterns, to a feeling of tightness and hardness and restricted breathing. There is also a widespread hypersensitivity to pressure, so that, for example, trousers or dresses press uncomfortably. Many sufferers experience numbness in and around the scar area or even an aversion to being touched in the affected area or to touch the spot themselves. In the body, the scar often leaves a feeling of being cut off or severed. Some people no longer feel that the affected body part belongs to them and is foreign.

2.3.2 Effects of Fascial Adhesions on the Body

In comparison to scar tissue, adhesions in the tissue overall remain more open to further changes in their structure. They react faster to applied three-dimensional tension impulses and are open to restructuring. These are the good news. We will come back to them later with appropriate exercises. However, after injuries, there are initially various restrictions of this complex sliding and layering system.

> **Recognizing the effects of adhesions**
> - Cut-offfeeling
> - Feeling unable to breathe into the abdomen or the surgical area
> - Feeling of tightness in the body
> - Pulling sensation during movements or at rest
> - Movement only possible with additional effort
> - Stiffness in the body that was not there before the operation
> - Lack of muscle activation
> - Targeted training of abdominal muscles, pelvic floor muscles does not have the desired effect
> - Yoga and maximum stretches increase pain and discomfort in the body
> - Emergence or intensification of chronic pain conditions and tensions in the rest of the body (shoulder pain, neck tension, headaches)
> - Chronic tensions that only temporarily improve with therapy/massage and then return
> - Chronic pelvic pain, sciatica—pain, blockages of the pelvic joints
> - Reduced mobility of the hip joints
> - Emergence of new blockages or frequent spraining of the spine

Compared to scar tissue, adhesions represent inflexible connections between the tissue layers deep into the body space. The result is a loss of tissue mobility. Specifically, this means that excessively healed adhesions cause impairments of smoothness due to thickened tissue fibers. This results in unpleasant tensile stresses. The growth of pain sensors and fine nerves into the adhesions can also make this tissue particularly sensitive or easily irritated. Last but not least, inflammatory processes and pain can also be triggered (Stöckl 2019). The collagen deposits that form in a mesh-like manner during the formation of adhesions can cause movement restrictions both locally and in the rest of the body. If muscles and large fascial systems are associated with the adhesions, the tensile stress is transferred to the corresponding movement system. Thus, adhesions in the arms can, for example, impair the mobility of finger flexor tendons (Willard 2014b).

The **effects** of adhesions in the different tissue layers are particularly evident in movement patterns, as this requires the ability of the tissue layers to shift. This becomes noticeable, for example, after abdominal operations: Especially during breathing, there is a feeling of tightness; deep abdominal breathing is not possible despite all attempts.

If the execution of a movement that includes the surgical area is restricted by adhesions, and/or only possible against resistance or with the aid of compensation patterns, this can manifest as pulling pain during movements. When adhesions affect the deep fascia, which is connected to the musculature, it often leads to the feeling of not being able to properly control certain muscles or certain areas. In targeted muscle training, such as that of the pelvic floor or the abdominal muscles, the desired results are then missing despite intensive training. The gained strength cannot be maintained on its own without continuous practice. This also applies to stretching exercises, such as in yoga, when the desired change is perceived as too slow, does not occur as expected, or possibly even causes pain.

New blockages in the musculoskeletal system can often be traced back to deep and pronounced adhesions. Until then, these were probably completely inconspicuous, as the body effectively compensated for the lack of mobility in the surgical area in everyday life with the help of the surrounding healthy, i.e., still movable, connective tissue over a long period of time. Affected individuals thus develop more or less pronounced corresponding evasive movements and patterns over time. In the end, there are often chronic tension and pain conditions, the cause of which lies unrecognized in the adhesions.

2.3.3 Effects of Adhesions in the Abdominal Cavity on the Body (see Fig. 2.4)

To better understand the effects of adhesions in the abdominal cavity on the body, one must know that the abdominal cavity is mechanically designed for maximum frictionless movement and shiftability. Only in this way can it guarantee the optimal function of the organs. The stomach, intestines, and bladder can loosely shift relative to each other, allowing them to fill and empty relaxedly; the uterus can also expand maximally during pregnancy. It uses several strategies for this. The abdominal membrane sac (medically: Peritoneum, marked orange in the illustration) corresponds with its area of about two square meters to the area of the skin. Special fasciae and ligaments ensure stable attachment of the organs and good supply of vessels and nerves. At the same time, they guarantee adequate information regarding

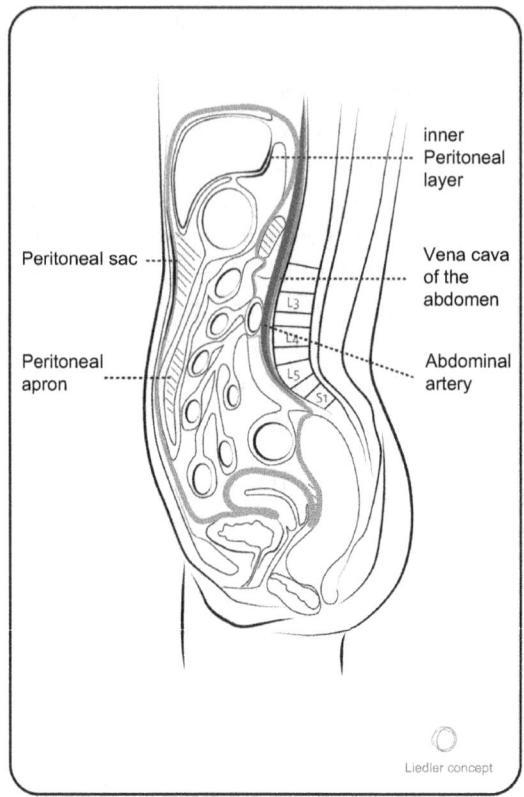

Fig. 2.4 Abdominal Membrane Sac. (© 2022 Liedler-Concept)

position, movement, and tension (Van Baal et al. 2016; Helsmoortel et al. 2002). The special nature of the abdominal membrane sac supports the frictionless shifting and movement of the organs relative to each other from the inside. How can one imagine this? Two sliding layers line the abdominal membrane sac from the inside and surround all organs. In contrast to the fine, web-like structure of the connective tissue that surrounds and permeates everything in the rest of the body to enable sliding and movement, the surface of the two sliding layers in the abdominal cavity is closed off by a special cell layer. This layer has the property that it does not bind or stick to other tissue layers when touched. This ensures minimal friction and maximum mobility of the organs. Additionally, there is a sliding fluid between these two tissue layers, which further reduces friction. In this way, relaxed, tension-free movement of the intestine and other organs is enabled (Van Baal et al. 2016).

If adhesions now form after surgery in the abdominal cavity (see Fig. 2.5), be it between the sliding surfaces in the abdominal cavity, between the organs themselves, or between organs and the abdominal wall, these create tension pulls. The tensions can unfavorably influence an entire body area, individual tissue layers, or even organs that are easily irritated.

This leads to a loss of mobility and flexibility due to the wound of the surgery, where restrictions form and cause a loss of mobility of the tissue layers and/or in relation to the organs. These connections can affect and disrupt organ movements, the movement and functionality of the intestines and sexual organs directly through the adhesions or indirectly through the increase in tension caused by the adhesions (Arung et al. 2011). Due to adhesions, changes in pelvic and organ positions can occur, which can complicate ultrasound diagnostics and the desire to have children and cause pain in the pelvic and hip area, e.g. through blockages of the pelvic joints (sacroiliac joints) or pelvic misalignments (Cheong et al. 2001). Many widespread symptoms are known, such as altered bowel activity, digestive problems up to intestinal obstruction or recurring bladder pain. Female patients describe pain during menstruation, ovulation or during sexual intercourse. Infertility, back pain, shoulder pain or chronic pelvic and sciatic pain are also mentioned in this context (Arung et al. 2011). From my own clinical experience, I can add the following symptoms to this list: shoulder and neck tension,

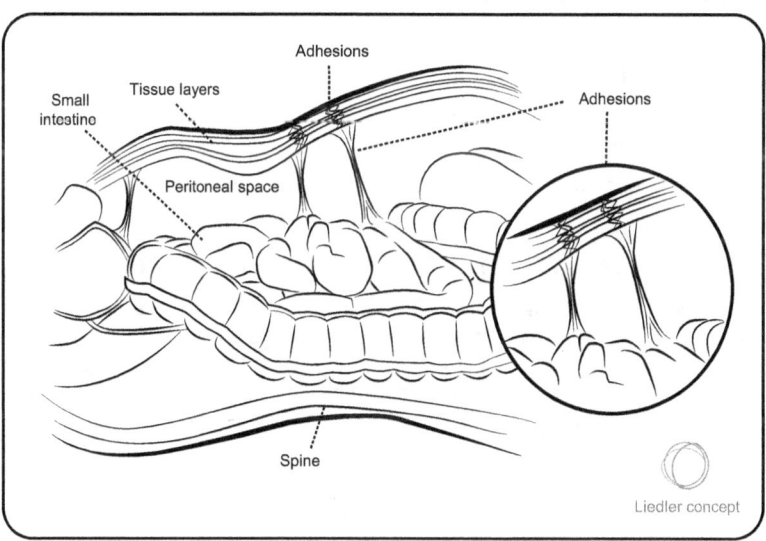

Fig. 2.5 Adhesions in the depth of the abdominal cavity. (© 2022 Liedler-Concept)

headaches, disc problems, temporomandibular joint blockages and pain, frequent and unexpected twisting of the spine, knee pain and other inexplicably occurring pain symptoms, for which little explanations and effective therapy suggestions are found in conventional medicine.

> **Identifying possible deep adhesions**
> - Altered bowel activity, irritable bowel, bloated abdomen, digestive problems, intestinal obstruction
> - Recurring bladder pain without inflammation
> - Pain during menstruation, ovulation and/or during sexual intercourse
> - Altered orgasmic ability
> - Infertility, problems getting pregnant
> - Back pain
> - Shoulder pain, neck tension, headaches
> - Chronic pelvic pain, sciatic pain, blockages of the pelvic joints
> - Unexpected frequent twisting of the spine
> - Reduced mobility of the hip joints
> - Knee pain, inflammation of the Achilles tendon
> - Swelling in the legs
> - Temporomandibular joint problems, problems with mouth opening

2.4 The Factor of Time—What Happens in the Body when the Scars are Old?

Scars, adhesions in the tissue and adhesions in the abdominal cavity are the best possible result of the wound healing process after a tissue injury. They come and if untreated, they stay. In the best case, they are optimally integrated by the body and it finds a new and good balance around them.

> **THE BODY ALWAYS MAKES THE BEST OF ITS POSSIBILITIES**
> Scar, adhesions in the tissue and in the abdominal cavity are normal consequences of a surgery and the healing process. They come and if untreated, they stay. The body adjusts and finds a new strategy and a new balance. Pain and restrictions occur when the body is overwhelmed and asks for help and support. Pain is NEVER without reason, but its language of overwhelm.

For this, our body uses many possibilities. Regardless of the point in life history when the scar and its companions are treated, the body restructures itself according to its possibilities. If no scar treatment is carried out, the original results of the wound healing process largely remain in the body. The body then provides the necessary compensations. Over time, these are possibly solidified or maintained in the system and the body does not function optimally, as described above. In old age, the experienced life stories accumulate, and the elasticity of the tissue decreases. The latter means that the body's possibilities to compensate for movement restrictions (adhesions, stress, life history etc.) are also reduced. How can this be imagined concretely using the example of an abdominal surgery?

Since large parts of the abdominal cavity are not designed to perceive pain (Struller et al. 2017), adhesions and stickiness in the abdominal cavity can initially remain completely symptomless. They are not perceived by the patient themselves. However, unnoticed, the original freedom of movement in the surgical area is altered by additional strands of tissue. The stiffness and tension of the tissue is locally increased by irritations and swellings. At the same time, the ingrowth of pain sensors into the adhesions leads to both increased stimulation of the nerves and a stronger sensitization. The adjacent tissue and muscles then transmit this new information to the environment and to adjacent bony structures. As a result, these changes can affect the internal balance of organs and alter the interplay of muscles, fasciae, bones (Tozzi et al. 2011). Through our muscles and our connective tissue, which both determine movement throughout the body, it may now be that this correction in the body system also transfers to distant parts of the body (Schleip et al. 2014). New movement patterns and protective postures emerge (Liedler 2020).

Let's look at the spine, for example: As a fixed component, it is responsible for our upright posture and statics. New overloading stimuli are forwarded, processed accordingly, and can result in deviations in movement and upright posture. For example, prolonged unilateral incorrect loading of the spine can lead to overloading and wear and tear on the opposite side, including the resulting pain (Pischinger 2010). If the body system is too overwhelmed, it may be that even normal stimuli result in excessive muscle tension and slowed body reaction.

With regard to our factor of time, one must also consider that humans become stiffer and less elastic with age. It therefore becomes increasingly difficult for him to compensate well for increased tension in the tissue (Pischinger 2010). This could lead to some scar tensions or protective postures only gaining significance years or decades after an operation due to this loss of elasticity and changes in the tissue or drying out in the sliding systems (Guimberteau et al. 2010). For the patient, this means that a previously unknown pain symptomatology arises in the body, as the body can no longer adequately compensate for the additional changes or traces that operations, scars, and adhesions leave permanently in the tissue.

2.4.1 Possibilities of Change

Basically, our body reacts very flexibly to life history and external influences. It constantly tries to establish the best possible balance at the moment.
Our body always makes the best of its possibilities. It is our best friend. If pain arises, there is a reason for it. Pain is stressful and strenuous for the mind and body. This is not a state that is voluntarily maintained. Thus, the body always strives for a pain-free and relaxed general state in its adaptation reactions.
The techniques of the Liedler Concept are based on this changeability and adaptation structure of the body. Because they specifically use the flexible abilities and properties of the connective tissue that the body uses to adapt to physical stimuli. Such as building up muscle in response to muscle training or reacting to stretching stimuli with better suppleness of the tissue (Schleip 2003a,b).

As part of the Liedler Concept, three-dimensional, rhythmically dynamic movements are incorporated into the sequence of LK self-application, as they occur in everyday life. In conjunction with targeted grip techniques, changes are made directly in the dense structure of scar and adhesion where the body is actually impaired (Liedler 2020). Rigid and dense tissue is broken down and at the same time the mobility and flexibility of the tissue is regained. The goal is to enable the body to return to its normal function and suppleness (Ingber 2008a).

At the same time, the release of lubricant is stimulated by movements, such as hyaluron or the fluid in the abdominal cavity. The latter maintains and promotes the relaxed sliding of the tissue layers. In this way, friction in the abdominal cavity and between the organs is reduced, the sliding between the tissue layers is supported (Van Baal et al. 2016). Through the connective tissue that connects us from head to toe, the gained lightness and the new movement expression are automatically transferred to the entire body system and chronic tensions decrease (Liedler 2017, 2020).

2.5 Tissue—Mechanical Influenceability of Adhesions in the Tissue and Adhesions in the Abdominal Cavity

Tissue responds to touch and stress. The body senses through special sensors in the skin. It responds to mechanical stress with an adaptation of the tissue. This creates the feeling of, for example, muscle soreness with new movements and new powerful demands. The muscles and all necessary tissue systems remodel and adapt. If these new movements are no longer needed, for example, if this specific sport is no longer performed, the body gradually reduces the strength and flexibility that was needed and gained. Only what is regularly brought is preserved. This is familiar to anyone who has ever had a cast and/or had to rest significantly. After the cast is removed or at the end of the immobilization, the muscles in this area are shrunken and weak, the body part even appears smaller.

Scar therapy and other manual therapies take advantage of this ability of the change: the special property of connective tissue to adapt and restructure itself specifically (Guimberteau and Armstrong 2016; Langevin et al. 2011). Scars, adhesions in the tissue, and adhesions in the abdominal cavity are also formed from connective tissue. It is therefore possible to influence and change these structures with appropriate manual stimuli. Here, the therapist and you yourself can achieve a lot.

What does this mean specifically? In general, connective tissue responds to mechanical stimuli, such as pressure or tension, with the activation of remodeling processes. This is used in treatments where tissue reorganizations are specifically provoked or freedom of movement and sliding layers are to be restored (Threlkeld 1992; Carano and Siciliani 1996). Remodeling processes are triggered, which subsequently break down and reshape "defective" parts of scars and adhesions (Liedler 2020).

In general, tissues and fasciae have a high density of sensors. They help to perceive mechanical forces and to assess them. Through special sensors for pressure and vibration, deep tensile, pressure, and shear stresses, the body recognizes fast and slow stimuli in the sense of a feedback system. As a result, it can then adjust and possibly reduce muscle tension (Schleip 2003a,b).

Depending on the respective stress, the components of the superficial and deep tissue layers react differently. In fact, the individual tissue fibers align themselves according to the movements and then return to their original position. A flexible and optimally deformable tissue structure made of fibers, mini bubbles, and sliding substances such as hyaluronic acid ensures smooth sliding to each other and enables the body to move and absorb and transmit occurring forces and tension. *"Even wide and fast displacements of tendons are possible without major resistance and without causing movement in the surrounding tissues."* (Guimberteau 2014, p. 106). In the depth of the body, dense tissue layers absorb the acting forces and transmit them to the associated body system (Trindade et al. 2012).

With regard to therapeutic treatment, studies have shown the possibility that densifications and thickening of the tissue layers can be influenced by manual interventions. For example, ultrasound has shown that after a physiotherapeutic treatment with manual tissue techniques, the thickness of the different tissue layers in the neck area could be reduced. This then also had a positive effect on accompanying chronic pain conditions in the patient (A. Stecco et al. 2014).

It is important that the intensity is individually adapted to the patient depending on the stage of the wound and wound healing phase during treatment and is gradually increased. Thus, in the initial stage of wound healing, gentle, soothing techniques and lymphatic drainage support wound closure and swelling reduction (Standley and Meltzer 2008). From day five after the surgery, painless, short moderate stretches promote the subsiding of inflammatory processes, the restoration of tissue balance, and the functional alignment of the tissue fibers. From day 21 of wound healing, the sensitive new tissue is gradually solidified and adapted according to the movements and stresses. Normal everyday stresses are now desired to promote the restoration of the strength and flexibility of the tissue. The stresses can now be individually adapted to the necessary need and gradually increased (Van den Berg 2014). In scar therapy according to the Liedler Concept, a precise fine-tuning of the duration and intensity of stretching and treatment techniques is essential to counteract an inappropriate or exaggerated formation of scar tissue. Through the remodeling and adaptation capabilities of the tissue, it is possible to influence adhesions and at the same time restore the normal sliding system in the connective tissue and a smooth power transmission in the body (Liedler 2020).

2.5.1 Old Scars—How Long can I still make Changes?

First and foremost, it should be said that the event of the surgery has a point in time when the scar, the adhesions in the tissue, and the adhesions in the abdominal cavity are formed. However, this does not mean that these structures are as old as the operation has passed. Instead, since the formation of the scar and the associated adhesions, all movement and force axes in the body are shaped and guided by the surgery and its consequences. This influence, which emanates from them, contributes to the general balance or imbalance (Arung et al. 2011). At the same time, our body is constantly subjected to regeneration and repair processes. This means that every cell in the body and every tissue component has a certain lifespan, then dies, is broken down and/or replaced by a new batch. Collagen, the main component of scars and adhesions, has a lifespan of about one to one and a half years until it is renewed (von Heymann and Stecco 2016). Our collagen is thus replaced, rebuilt or degraded as the acting tension states and the surrounding tissue condition require. To summarize: Our body has the ability to respond to mechanical stimuli from the outside and accordingly change the movement information in the tissue. Manual therapy and LK take advantage of exactly this ability. So there is ALWAYS, regardless of how old the scar is, the possibility to positively influence rigid tissue structures after surgery.

> **Important**
> The time since the surgery does not correspond to the age of the scar tissue! The surgery has a date and thus a point in time.
> Scars and adhesions consist of collagen, which is constantly renewed at least every one to one and a half years.
> The scar and adhesion structures are therefore a maximum of 1.5 years old and can be influenced and changed anew at ANY time.

2.6 Scars as Part of Life History (Understanding—Physically and Mentally)

A scar will always be a part of one's own life history. Even if one would perhaps like to forget and undo the experience that led to it. The traces remain visible on the skin. But also inside the body, lasting traces are left.

Objectively viewed, there is hardly a greater physical boundary violation than a surgery. Even if the decision for a surgery is usually made in consensus and with consent or out of a life-threatening situation, the incision means opening the body and thus the maximum crossing of one's own body boundary. A surgery is the intrusion into the body's interior. It leaves a wound or a tissue defect that must heal afterwards.

For a good conclusion of the surgery or the deep injury, it is therefore necessary to heal physically and to restore the body's well-being from the surface to the depth—in the sense of a soft permeable elasticity, flexibility, and mobility—as best as possible. How can you achieve this? The focus here is primarily on the permeability of movement and the suppleness in all axes of movement. This simultaneously results in the pain sensors being freed from the compressions, subsequently being less or no longer activated, and not reminding us painfully of the event with every movement. At the same time, it is also about mentally understanding and processing the experience. Only in this way will it ultimately become an accepted and "peaceful" part of life history. Specifically, this means consciously understanding what has happened and that the event is OVER. That is, the date in time at which it took place had a beginning and an end and is therefore now located in the past. "Mentally peaceful" then also means that touching and moving the scar is possible in a relaxed manner and without emotional excitement, restlessness, or reluctance (Van der Kolk 2015).

Understanding Scars as Part of Life History Understanding here means, on the one hand, mentally understanding and realizing that the event is over and in the past. And on the other hand, getting to know oneself physically anew, understanding the changes through scar and adhesion, and understanding that everything has healed well. In this way, the experience of the surgery can become a peaceful and relaxed part of life history as a completed event.

2.6.1 Physical Healing

Every major wound leaves physical changes: the superficial scar and the deeper adhesions in the tissue or strands deep in the abdominal cavity and a changed perception and experience of the affected area. The brain is constantly informed about the changed movement dynamics via nerves and pain sensors in the tissue. Protective postures and compensation mechanisms are "automatically" created with every movement using the information sensors in the connective tissue. The goal of the body is to make the execution of every movement as easy and smooth as possible. This works because the supple connective tissue surrounding the affected area has almost infinite possibilities to extend to compensate for the tight, rigid adhesion strands. In this way, movement can flow relatively unnoticed through the body, despite adhesions. However, from a certain degree, these hardened and compacted tension lines are so strong that they activate nerves and are then perceived as pain in the brain. More often, however, despite the adhesions, the nerve stimulus remains so low that it is not perceived as acutely painful in the brain. Nevertheless, the body must compensate for the tension lines and changes. In the worst case, this goes well until the tissue and fascial compensation system collapses and chronic pain occurs due to permanent overload in other areas of the body (Gold and Gebhart 2010).

> From physical to mental comprehension
>
> - Through the physical understanding of the scar with the help of LK self-exercises, the optical and tangible changes can be experienced and possibly also changed.
> - Touching the scar and the affected tissue and area also opens up the space for the mental understanding of what has happened.

2.6.2 Mental Comprehension

In order to process a surgery well and to classify the experience as part of the past, it is important to also process it mentally well. Since the brain reacts differently in stress situations than normal, this is often not easy.

Mental, relaxed experience of a surgery
The mental experience of an operation is processed in the best case without agitation. This is achieved by creating a safe space, through sufficient clarification and a professional, warm accompaniment of the responsible team. Touching and/or therapy of the scar and the affected restrictions after the surgery can take place in such a case relaxed and without major emotional waves. The change of the tissue is classified as a new experience, experienced and the scar is quietly integrated into the body. The experience can be consciously perceived as ONE past PART of the life story (Van der Kolk 2015).

Traumatic experience of a surgery
An operation with and without complications can, however, also be experienced very traumatically by the affected person and accordingly poorly processed.

> **Recognition of a traumatic mental experience**
> - Ignoring the scar
> - Not being able to touch the scar.
> - Not allowing others to touch it.
> - Discomfort when looking at or touching the scar.
> - Horror of the scar
> - Not wanting or being able to talk about the operation.
> - Having no words for it.
> - When approaching the healed, closed scar, it is emotionally and vividly experienced in the mind like an open wound.
> - When talking about the surgery, when touching the scar, unpleasant feelings arise such as: powerlessness, fear, dizziness, nausea, a woolly, foggy feeling in the head.

What is happening here in our brain? In concrete terms, this means that the brain activates our survival strategies and releases stress hormones. If the experience is overpowering and the self-experience of powerlessness dominates, in the worst case, the brain shuts down the part of our brain responsible for the conscious processing of the experience. This brain region is anatomically located behind the forehead and is called the prefrontal cortex. It is responsible for making detailed and accurate observations in a situation, consciously perceiving experiences from different perspectives, and thus creating a complex picture of the situation in order to then make the best approach or decision. From all this information, a memory is then created that has a BEGINNING and an END, which can be located on the timeline of our life story in the past. However, if there is a massive overload in a situation, the prefrontal cortex is completely or partially deactivated via a reflex-like reaction of the nervous system. This leads physically to a protective reaction in the sense of freezing, to avoid potential injuries, to a reduced perception of pain, and to a reduced heart rate and breathing. The body reacts, but analytical thinking is no longer possible: large parts of conscious perception are partially or completely switched off. In this mode, therefore, no end of the experience is perceived. The experience of the trauma and the fear remains time-independent and real and cannot be located in the past. In this sense, individual components of the experience, such as the scar, can become triggers that, for example, when touched, trigger the complete alarm reaction just as if it were part of the now and not part of a memory. The primary reaction is then fear with the corresponding physical reactions. Even when the trigger has subsided, the body still takes longer to restore relaxation and balance the nervous system (Van der Kolk 2015).

Physical effects of a traumatic experience of surgery
Unprocessed Traumas leave tension in the tissue. This tension can also change towards reduced tissue mobility. Even if the nervous system regulates itself again after surgery, a sensitization, inhibition, or a complete aversion associated with the scar may remain. Touching the scar becomes a major challenge, accompanied by discomfort, it is avoided to think about the event etc. Often the surgical area is simply excluded from the body image and forgotten. In everyday life, such a scar is then coupled with emotional discomfort, with fear, a threatening feeling, or also with symptoms such as nausea, a "foggy" head, horror before or during touch, rejection of touch, feeling cut off. Over time, this subtle constant state of alert, coupled with the release of stress factors in the body and the lack of relaxation of the nervous system, then leads to the development of chronic diseases such as nonspecific pain in the neck area, migraines, digestive problems or irritable bowel or asthma (Van der Kolk 2015).

With the help of physical work with the scar and a trained, compassionate therapist, as well as with the help of LK self-exercises, as described in this book, it is possible to approach the story and leave this fear and tension mode behind again. *"A real change can only take place when the body learns that the danger is over and it lives again in the present reality."* (Van der Kolk 2015, p. 32).

In order to experience a peaceful state and a relaxed body feeling with the scar and the associated process, it is important to be able to feel comfortable both mentally and emotionally and physically in the own body again. So it's about being able to move smoothly, stress and physically demand without pain, but at the same time also about being able to experience touch relaxed. The big goal is to integrate the scar as a completed part of our life story into our life.

References

Asmussen, Peter D., Brigitte Söllner. 2010. Die Prinzipien der Wundheilung. Bd. Sonderausgabe. Embrach: Kammerlander.
Gold, M. S., G. F. Gebhart. 2010. „Nociceptor sensitization in pain pathogenesis". Nature Medicine 16 (11): 1.248–57.
Heymann, Wolfgang von, Carla Stecco. 2016. „Fasziale Dysfunktionen". *Manuelle Medizin* 54: 303–6. https://doi.org/10.1007/s00337-016-0172-1.

Langevin, H. M., J. R. Fox, C. Koptiuch, G. J. Badger et al. 2011. „Reduced thoracolumbar fascia shear strain in human chronic low back pain". BMC Musculoskeltal Disorders 12 (203): 1–11.

Liedler, Michaela. 2017. „Einfluss von postoperativen Adhäsionen nach Sektio auf chronischen Low Back Pain – eine Pilotstudie". Masterthese, Krems: DUK.

———. 2020. *„Peritoneale Adhäsionen – Fasziale Behandlung nach dem Liedler-Konzept"*. Berlin, Heidelberg: Springer Verlag GmbH.

Van den Berg, F. 2014. „Die Physiologie der Faszie". Lehrbuch Faszien, herausgegeben von R. Schleip, T. W. Findely, L. Chaitow, P. A. Huijing, 1. Auflage, 110–14. München: Elsevier GmbH.

Van der Kolk, B.A. 2015. Verkörperter Schrecken: Traumaspuren in Gehirn, Geist und Körper und wie man sie heilen kann. Lichtenau: G. B. Probst Verlag.

3

The Basics of the Liedler Concept (LK)

The focus of the Liedler techniques is to specifically influence scars and adhesions in superficial and deep tissue layers as well as adhesions in the abdominal cavity down to the **deep layers**. Remodeling processes are activated and the tissue sliding layers are **permanently** restored. This creates the conditions for the body to maintain this freedom of movement in the long term.

In order to be able to carry out the self-exercises effectively, the basic principles of the Liedler concept (LK) are explained. What exactly is it about? What is the idea behind it and what is to be achieved or what can be achieved through the self-application of the manual Liedler techniques? This chapter describes the therapeutic approach with its basic principles and the different treatment levels and goals of the concept. Differences to other scar therapies are highlighted and it is shown what is actually different or special about this current approach to the treatment of adhesions in the tissue and adhesions in the abdominal cavity. The focus is on self-efficacy and the question of when to start with the LK self-exercises.

Locally, the tissue changes are often noticeable as unpleasant or sensitive nodules, hardenings and compactions that can trigger pulling in the tissue during movement. In the rest of the body, more or less noticeable protective postures often arise, which are frequently associated with

---

Supplementary Information The electronic version of this chapter contains additional material, which can be accessed via the following link https://doi.org/10.1007/978-3-662-68482-5_3. The videos can be played by clicking on the **DOI link** in the legend of a corresponding figure, or by scanning this link with the SN More Media App.

chronic tension and pain conditions. Even if the connection is not immediately apparent from the outside, there are invisible connections that can be quickly, efficiently and permanently positively influenced with the Liedler concept. The suppleness of the compacted tissue is increased, promoted or regained through movements. This makes protective postures unnecessary and chronic pain conditions, which are related to the consequences of the operation, improve and/or disappear completely. Since skin, connective tissue and muscles can be influenced and changed by mechanical stimuli such as stretching, pulling and pressure stimuli, self-treatment becomes possible. This can increase local blood circulation, improve cell metabolism and at the same time relax the muscles. Pain can be alleviated and fear in this context can be let go (Moyer et al. 2004).

3.1 Therapeutic Approach—Idea and Goal of LK Self-Exercises

The body represents a movable system. To maintain this flexibility, it is always in motion. Even during sleep, the tissue is subtly and gently rocked by the respiratory and organ movements. The Liedler Concept aims to restore the original flexibility in the surgical area and thus in the body. The goal is for the body to be able to move freely in all directions despite the scar and to perform sports or other stresses without tension.

Through the LK techniques and the LK-self-exercises the tissue receives impulses and stimuli, in response to which the adhesions are again dismantled and broken down. Specifically, the aim is to stimulate the firm, immobile tissue strands in the superficial and deep tissue layers caused by the surgery to change back into soft, flexible, and dynamic structures. As a result, the tissue layers can slide against each other again, and relaxation occurs in the affected area and throughout the body. As a result, chronic tensions in the shoulders, back, head, and jaw joint decrease or disappear entirely. Last but not least, the breath can again expand into the affected areas of the body, leading to better relaxation. Although working with the scar and adhesions can be painful and may feel sore afterwards, the LK self-exercises do not provoke a wound with excessive inflammatory processes in the tissue, but on the contrary, initiate a moderate tissue remodeling. The changes and increasing mobility achieved through the LK techniques are then automatically incorporated into the existing movement system. Practical experience has also shown that the gained flexibility is maintained in the long term and permanently incorporated into the body system.

> For all those who have already tried many therapies at this point: There are many sliding layers at different depths and between tissue layers that want to be released to regain the maximum body comfort. With scars and adhesions, patience and perseverance are often required for the corresponding success. Regular use of the LK self-exercises helps to make compacted tissue layers flexible again step by step. **Every gained sliding layer remains a gained sliding layer in the body and a step towards lightness!** It does **not** re-adhere!

The LK therapy specifically targets the following points:

- Local remodeling of scar tissue and adhesions in the tissues and abdominal area from rigid, inflexible to soft, harmonious, deformable structures
- Restoring or improving the sliding surfaces and sliding properties in the connective tissue between the superficial and deep tissue layers to increase flexibility
- Restoring or improving the sliding surfaces in the abdominal area to reduce tension in the abdominal area and allow the organs to move again relaxed or function optimally again
- Mobilization of the adhered tissue layers so that the tissue can be better supplied and swellings in the tissue decrease and disappear faster

Scars and adhesions and their influence on the body can be tested and then treated using the LK scar test (see Sect. 3.5). Restrictions in relation to surrounding joints and movement axes can be made visible and tangible. Protective postures and compensation mechanisms can be positively influenced and resolved through the self-exercises. In doing so, **everyone** can take advantage of the body's ability to restore elasticity, mobility, and flexibility in the tissue (Dodd et al. 2006; Liedler 2020). As a result, the LK self-treatment supports and facilitates the integration of scars and adhesions locally into the affected area and globally into the body system (Liedler 2017, 2020).

3.2 When to Delay Self-Exercises

Generally, the acute wound healing processes are always a sensitive phase in which the scar should be handled very carefully. The primary goal is to ensure that the wound and the underlying tissue layers heal well. This applies especially to the first 14 days of wound healing. During this time, heavy loads, pressure, tension or shifting loads on the fresh scar should be avoided in order to achieve a good wound closure of the superficial skin and tissue layers (Van den Berg 2014). This also means that powerful direct techniques that would promote the separation of the wound are prohibited in this initial wound healing phase. They would increase the inflammatory processes and could thus delay wound healing (Fourie 2014). Normally, the crust detaches itself as soon as the wound is closed and can be considered an indicator of successful skin repair. However, it should be noted here that tissue regeneration reaches its peak after six to 16 days and the maximum strength of the new tissue is sometimes only regained weeks later (Asmussen and Söllner 2010; Bordoni 2023).

In the case of an acute inflammation or open areas in the scar area, it is urgently necessary to wait with the LK self-exercises. Inaccurate treatment at too early a stage and exceeding one's own limits must be absolutely avoided. The basic rule is **always** and for every technique, that the intensity precisely chosen and work with the body must be done with care and mindfulness.

- As long as the wound is still healing, it is URGENT: NO pulling apart of the wound
- NO heavy load on the wound with pressure or tension
- NO muscle training
- NO lifting and carrying of heavy things

3.3 Setting the Right Focus and Using Two Basic Principles

Many scar therapies focus only on the externally visible scar. However, the size of the wound under the skin in the tissue layers is usually much larger (see Fig. 3.1). During healing, it leaves adhesions and thus significant changes in the body and sliding layers of the tissue.

LK-Focus
Now, the goal of the LK self-exercises is to break down this invisible, dense, often immobile field of adhesions under the surface into small parts that can be mobile again. ***Each of these parts stands for a single LK focus.***

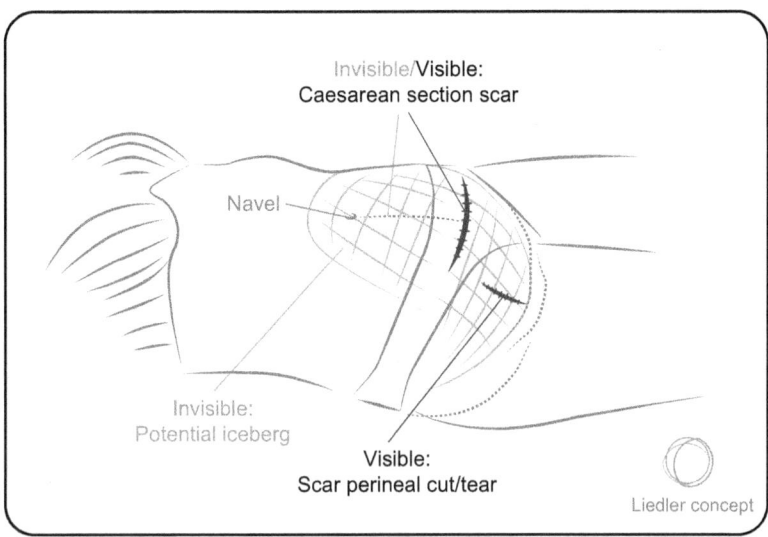

Fig. 3.1 Iceberg model of scar, tissue adhesion and adhesions in the abdominal area after cesarean section or perineal injury. (©2022 Liedler-Concept)

> If the iceberg under the skin is so large, why don't those affected recognize it earlier? The reason for this lies in the almost infinite mobility of healthy connective tissue. Although there are a multitude of adhesions in the surgical field, these are embedded in normally smooth and flexible connective tissue all around. The body uses this to compensate for the existing movement restrictions of adhesions and glued sliding layers. Therefore, a ***precise LK focus*** is needed in the LK self-applications to filter out the adhesions. With this, it is possible to perceive and feel adhesions where they are specifically located.

The LK focus is therefore on the deep adhesions **below** the scar (see Fig. 3.2). But how can these be identified? This involves sensing the tissue resistance at the end of the mobility. The focus of the LK technique is not on the scar surface, but is directed at a point in the deep tissue layers below the scar. This point is where no further mobility is possible in depth and a **hard** boundary becomes noticeable, which is always uncomfortable or painful. This corresponds to the end of the mobility of the skin **and** the underlying connective tissue layers in the iceberg.

Basically, every tissue has the property of being able to be moved up to a point before a noticeable movement boundary is reached (see Fig. 3.3).

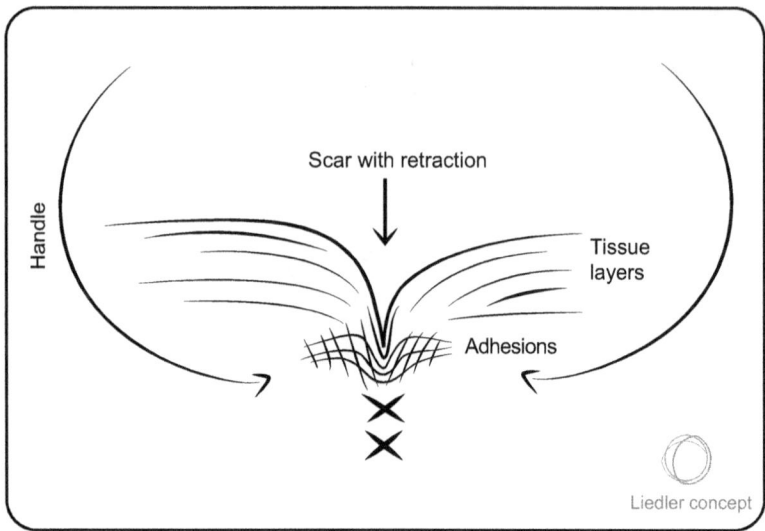

Fig. 3.2 LK focus on the deep layer BELOW the visible scar. (© 2022 Liedler-Konzept)

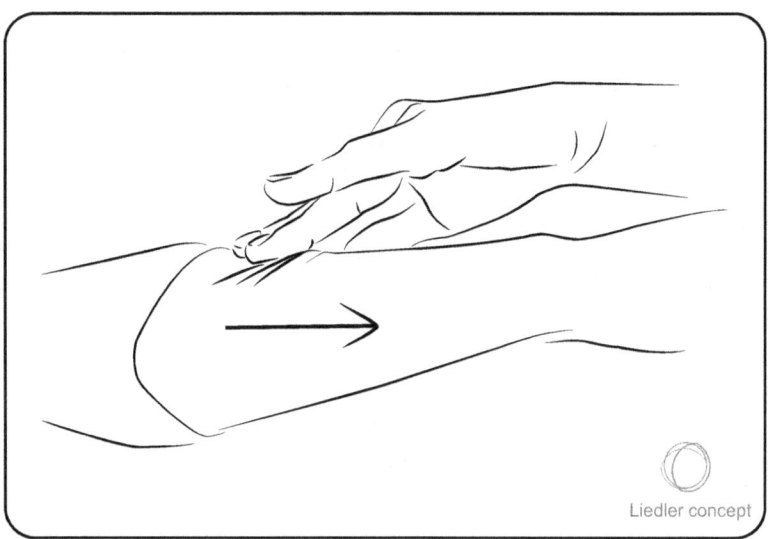

Fig. 3.3 Sensing the tissue boundary via tensile stress. (© 2023 Liedler-Konzept)

What does this movement boundary feel like in healthy, mobile tissue? Here's a small exercise: Take good contact with the skin with your entire fingertips, for example on the forearm or on the stomach. Move the skin

without sliding over the skin. The point at which you notice that your fingers begin to slide over the skin indicates the movement boundary of the tissue. Here, the end of mobility (tissue barrier) is reached. In the best case, you can see that wrinkles or small wrinkles form on the skin in the direction of movement.

In healthy, flexible connective tissue, this movement boundary (without loosing the precise skin contact and sliding over it!) feels painless, soft, elastic, and slightly springy (Levin 2014). Even when the skin's movement seems to come to an end, it is still possible to perform movements with the adjacent joints despite fixation. Tissue health therefore means that joints are still mobile even when the surrounding skin and tissue are put under tension.

> The elasticity and flexibility of **healthy tissue** is a prerequisite for our body to provide movement and a functioning body system despite many external influences, stresses, and restrictions. With the help of this suppleness of the tissue, superficial and deep adhesions can also be compensated to a certain extent if necessary. Despite the mentioned restrictions, enough mobility can still be provided.

Adhesions in the tissue and in the abdominal cavity change this elastic suppleness. The movement boundary or the end of mobility now feels abrupt, hard, inelastic, and often painful (Fourie 2014). If this movement boundary persists, the adjacent structures and joints are permanently restricted in their range of motion. As long as the skin is maximally displaced and held fixed, any movement then triggers an unpleasant to painful pulling sensation in the affected area.

By consciously blocking the existing mobility of skin and tissue by moving to the tissue boundary, it becomes very specifically possible to recognize and feel the actual impairment and effect of scar and adhesions on our movements.

LK Principle 1—Depth through Pretension
The first Principle 1 of the LK explains how you can reach and treat the deep tissue layers. Many common therapy approaches massage the scar tissue with pressure until it becomes soft again. Superficial lumps and densifications can also be well altered in this way. However, adhesions in the depth of the tissue and in the abdominal cavity cannot be reached with pressure impulses.

The LK therefore uses the fact that the deep tissue layers, which are freely movable or can slide under normal conditions, are connected to each other after surgery due to adhesions that have formed. In therapy, we want to restore the missing and inadequate suppleness and thus support the separation of these layers from each other. That means, it is about recognizing, dissolving, and treating adhesions individually.

Through the first LK principle, adhesion chains are created down to the depth of the abdominal cavity. The tissue layers are stretched apart like an accordion through pretensionin the tissue with the basic grip of the LK techniques, the so-called "scoop grip" (see Sect. 4.3) (see Fig. 3.4).

When the tissue layers are now put under tension, the adhesions between the layers are pulled apart and like an accordion, the pull is then passed on to the deeper layers. Wherever there are connections through adhesions, the pull is then passed on to the adjacent and underlying layers. So it's not just a single layer that is stretched, but the entire adhesion chain down to the depth that is connected to it. As a result, the restriction in the affected area initially intensifies and the actual impairment caused by the scar and the adhesions becomes concretely noticeable.

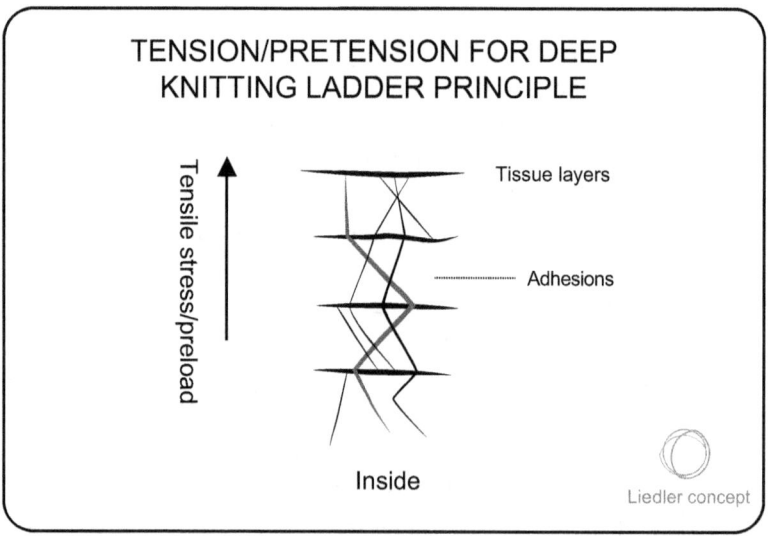

Fig. 3.4 Rope Ladder Principle—pretension for stretching the adhesion chain. (© 2022 Liedler Concept)

Using the LK focus, it is thus possible to directly target the adhesion and reach and treat the entire adhesion chain through the pretension. If the connection of the adhesion chain extends over the abdominal wall and subsequent adhesions into the abdominal cavity, it is also possible to influence deep-seated adhesions that affect mobility (adhesion chain into the abdominal cavity—see Fig. 2.5).

LK Principle 2—Fixed Point—Mobile Point
Now that the specific LK focus has been discussed in relation to the the first LK principle, the adhesion chain can be spanned down to the depth, and the second LK principle is now applied. I refer to it as "Fixed Point—Mobile Point". Why? In a first step, the adhesion chain must first be well fixed (**Fixed Point**). Subsequently, the movement impulse is then actively introduced into the tissue (**Mobile Point**), to change the adhesions towards suppleness and glide (see Fig. 3.5).

Creating a Fixed Point:
The goal is to establish a fixed point to enhance the LK focus on the adhesions in the desired area. First, these are brought under tension by

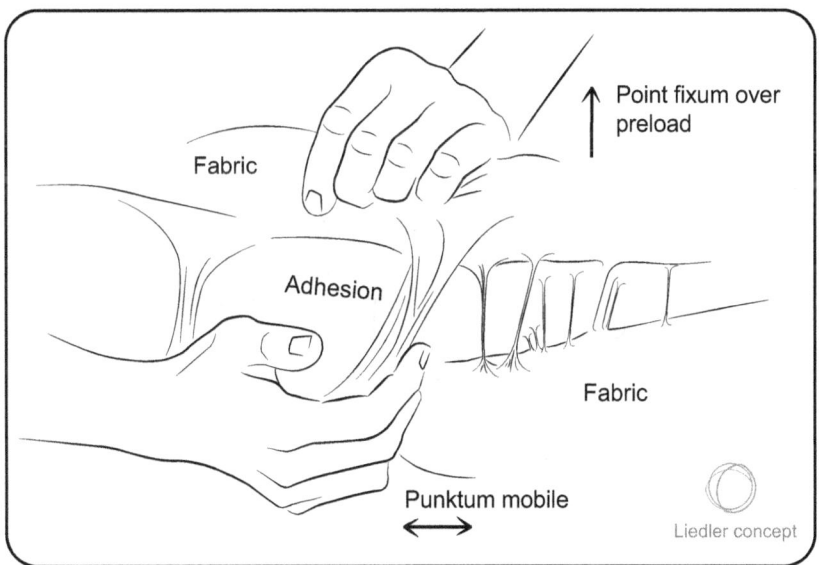

Fig. 3.5 Fixed Point—Mobile Point. (© 2022 Liedler Concept)

pre-tension (LK focus and first LK principle). They are then fixed using a scoop grip (see Fig. 3.7). This fixation ensures that the surrounding still movable connective tissue is largely switched off in this area. It is important that the fixed point is **always kept under constant tension** or **under tension** during the entire technique!

Creating a Mobile Point:
The task of the Mobile Point is to provoke movement exactly where movement is no longer possible due to adhesions in the area of the fixed point. Through mindful, slowly rhythmic rocking movements, movement impulses are set that lovingly expand the existing boundaries.

Therapeutic Movement Impulse of the Mobile Point (see Fig. 3.6)
The movement range of the Mobile Point goes from the tissue barrier (more precisely LK focus!) away a bit OVER the tissue boundary and back TO the barrier.

I recommend that you choose a specific movement and perform it SLOWLY, rhythmically and repetitively until the maximum range of motion is reached again. You can also orient yourself to the movements of the joints that are closest to the scar (e.g., circling the hip, pelvis, arms). In the

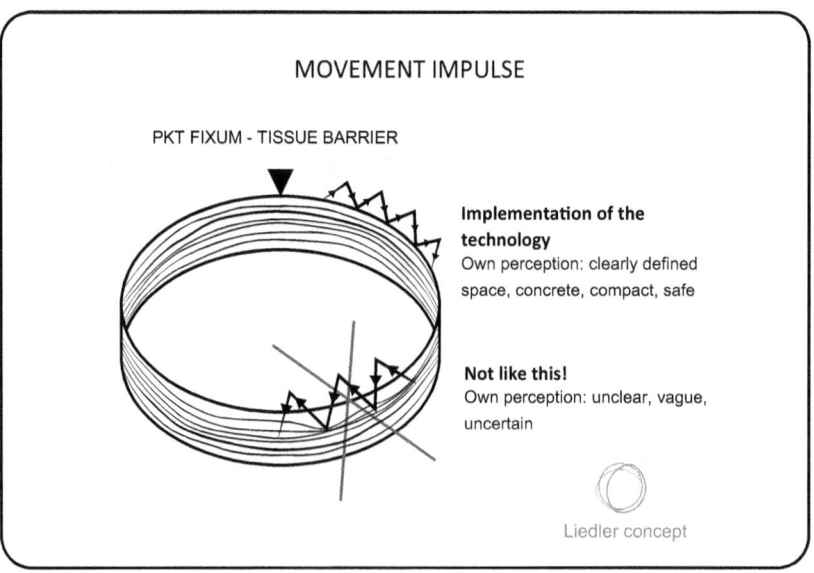

Fig. 3.6 Therapeutic movement impulse of change. (© 2022 Liedler Concept)

latter case, the large joints, with a continuously increasing movement, are slowly and mindfully moved through until the maximum range of motion is restored. The goal is to maximally increase the sliding layers and movement boundaries of the affected tissue and area that are restricted by the adhesions.

3.4 The Scoop Grip

The **scoop grip** is the basic grip of all LK techniques and LK self-exercises. With its help, the tensioning of the tissue layers down to the depth of the body is achieved. Even though it sounds simple and logical in theory, it takes some practice to learn the technique at first.

> **Instructions for the scoop grip (see Fig. 3.7)**
> For the execution, make good contact with the skin using your fingertips. Initially, keep your fingers extended. Then distort or shift the skin with your **extended** fingers until they almost start to slip over the skin. Now you have found the limit of the skin and tissue's mobility. If this limit is caused by adhesions, it now feels hard, inelastic, uncomfortable, pulling, or even painful. Please maintain this tension while you open your hand and thumb wide to cover as much skin as possible. Then make contact with the skin with your thumb and also shift the skin towards the fingers until the end of mobility. A fold begins to form between the fingers and thumb. It is important that no direct vertical pressure is applied into the depth, but the skin is "only" diagonally shifted or distorted. If you have kept your fingers extended as mentioned initially, you can now bend your fingertips and firmly enclose the fold (pinching sensation, hold and fix the tension (Punctum fixum).
>
> Make sure that both the fingers among themselves and the index fingers and thumbs of both hands touch each other. The fold between the fingers can be as large as possible. The smaller the fold, the more difficult it is to fix the adhesions (down to the depth of the iceberg).

> Dose the scoop gripso that you can hold it well. If necessary, use a paper towel or your T-shirt for assistance. The less you slide the scoop grip over the skin, the clearer the grip and the faster you will feel the improvement.

> The adhesion chains into the depth are achieved exclusively through the principle of pre-tension. Experience shows that at the beginning you might automatically apply pressure and press into the depth to get there. However, this causes the tissue layers to approach each other and the adhesions are no longer

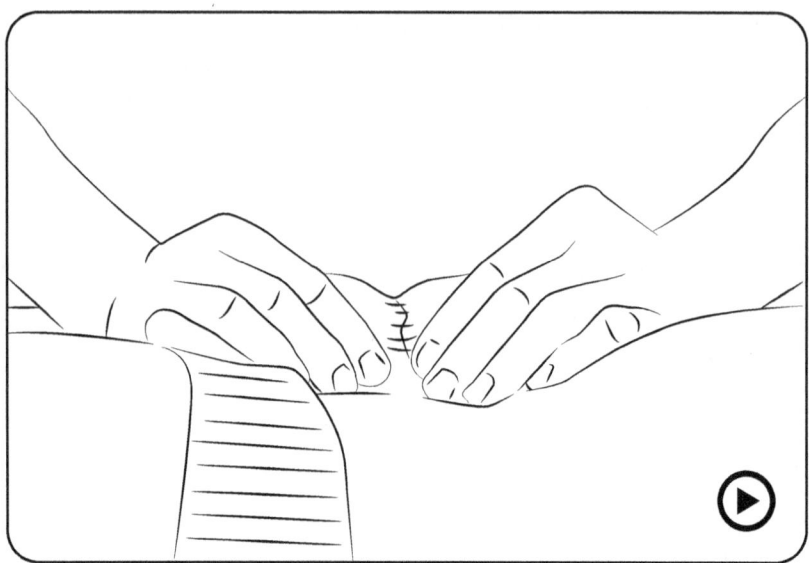

Fig. 3.7 scoop grip. (© 2023 Liedler-Concept ▸ https://doi.org/10.1007/000-fs3)

tensioned, but mix loosely with the other tissue layers. So you feel "some" tension in the tissue, but you do not get clear information about the adhesions and can no longer reach them specifically to the depth.

When you form a skin fold with the scoop grip, let it become larger rather than smaller! The more you feel that the skin fold is slipping away, the larger you need to grip the skin fold.

Entire Process of the Technique—The More Precise, the More Successful, the More Relaxed

About : The LK focus, the LK principles and the scoop grip make it possible to focus deep adhesions so that they can be treated and changed.

The exact process of the technique is important for success!

Instructions for the Process of the Technique
Start with the scoop grip (Punctum fixum). Using it as a starting point, you make the restrictions noticeable and visible: There is tension and a pull that is noticeably triggered by the adhesions. Both must now be kept constant

> throughout the entire process of the technique. In the next step, you want to perceive occurring changes. To do this, you introduce a movement impulse into the body via the Punctum mobile. This impulse stimulates the adhesions to remodel exactly where restrictions are present. Attention: Since pain sensors, which have grown into the adhesions during wound healing, are now irritated, the intensity increases initially and it can be perceived as painful. So be careful! However, through the continuous movement and expansion of the movement (Punctum mobile), the constricted layers begin to glide again, the movement gradually increases. And little by little, the feeling of tension and the pain slowly subside.

End of the Technique In practice, it is often at this very moment that a deep breath is taken. That is, only at this moment does the actual relaxation in body and mind occur. For this reason, it is absolutely important to always carry out the LK self-exercises until this point of relaxation. End here means that the freedom of movement is restored as much as possible **and** the intensity and the pain have decreased by at least two-thirds compared to the beginning.

> The LK self-exercises are derived directly from everyday life and should be incorporated exactly there. Especially when it pulls, when any movement becomes noticeably noticeable or a chronic state of tension reminds you that the iceberg in the body still represents too tight a corset. Each clearly executed application of the LK self-exercise brings about a liberation. Each sliding layer that is restored is a won sliding layer.

3.5 Identifying Restrictions with the Scar Check of the Liedler Concept

Before going into the different levels of scar treatment, I would like to briefly introduce the special scar check of the Liedler Concept. The LK-scar test is essentially the diagnostic basis and concrete starting point of each treatment or self-exercise.

You had surgery and want to know if the scar is affecting your body, restricting or disturbing movements? Sometimes the consequences of scars and adhesions in the tissue and in the abdominal area are so prominent that you are reminded of them by unpleasant feelings, pain and radiations. In the affected area, something is different and it is especially not yet good. However, it may also be that your body compensates and balances the accompanying adhesions so well that the scar appears inconspicuous and seemingly has no effects on the body. In some cases, the effects of scar and adhesions do not show obviously where the surgery took place, but through chronic tension or pain conditions in other areas of the body.

Even if adhesions often remain undiagnosed, the LK scar test offers the possibility to make real effects and restrictions of scar and adhesions noticeable and visible—clear and unequivocal. The LK scar test can be directed to the superficial or deep layers or specific joints or noticeable movements in relation to the area of surgery and can be tested specifically. The subsequent treatment immediately improves the feeling of well-being in the body and a feeling of lightness returns, see Fig. 3.8.

3.5.1 Check of the Superficial Layers

The superficial layers concern the visible scar plus the tissue layers directly adjacent to it. If the scar heals well, it will visually turn white and can be easily moved in relation to the adjacent tissue layers in all directions up to an elastic end of movement. The aim is always to explore the entire range of movement in one direction—i.e., to move as far as possible.

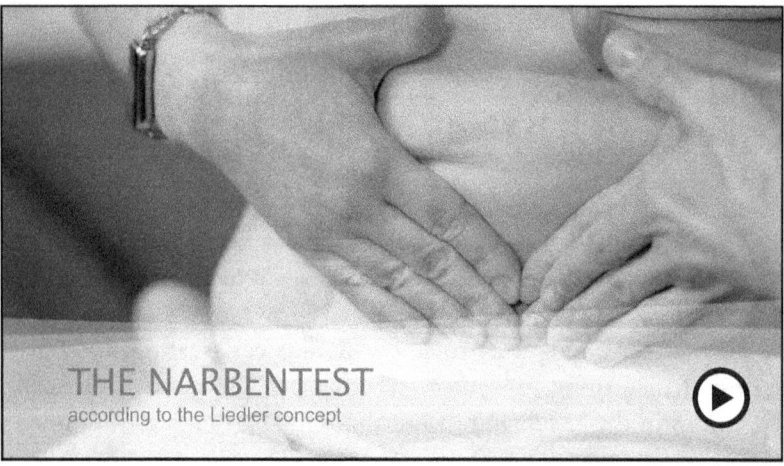

Fig. 3.8 The LK scar test. (▸ https://doi.org/10.1007/000-fs2)

> **Implementation of the LK scar test for the superficial layers**
>
> For the test of the superficial layers, establish good contact with the fingertips on one side of the scar and then carefully and lovingly move the skin layers as far as possible in one direction. At a certain point, you reach the end of movement, namely where you would start to slide with your fingers over the skin with further movement. How does this end feel? Is it elastic or does it feel hard and inelastic? You may also notice lumps or nodules under the skin.
>
> To explore the end of movement even more clearly, you can now increase the push with your fingers a little more—without sliding over the skin. Does the unpleasant feeling intensify? Does a pulling sensation or other unusual skin sensations appear?

> If you are unsure which tissue quality feels "normal", test a spot without a scar.

Evaluation

If the end of movement is soft, elastic, movable and feels inconspicuous, this means that the tissue layers are well movable relative to each other and that there are no adhesions there.

However, if the end of movement is hard, firm, inelastic and unpleasant, then the tissue is adhered. If the unpleasant feeling intensifies during the check and the hardness also increases, then this is a clear indication of dense adhesions of the scar and the adjacent layers. The next step would then be the implementation of an LK treatment e.g. with local techniques (see Figs. 4.10 and 4.11).

3.5.2 Examination of the Deep Layers

Normally movable tissue layers move easily and with low friction to each other. This allows movement and protects the body. Mechanical forces, such as pressure or tensile stress, which act on the skin, are absorbed by the mobility of the tissue and are transmitted in such a way that they cannot cause damage in depth and organs remain unburdened. As soon as tissue layers are glued together by a healing process, this suppleness is restricted. Specifically, this means that pressure and tensile stresses are transmitted deeper into the body and there are real restrictions in the interaction between muscles and the surrounding tissue structures. Organ movements can also be irritated by this. The consequences include feelings of tightness in the body, the feeling of not being able to breathe deeply, or also radiating tensions that usually appear during movement or can also manifest in the fact that muscles can no longer be controlled accordingly. This means, you train, but do not experience the corresponding training effect.

To detect these deep adhesions, the fact is used that adhesions span between tissue layers and connect them to each other. If these tissue layers are now tensioned with tensile stress, the entire adhesion chain can be brought into tension down to the depth. You can then clearly and concretely perceive and feel this.

> **Implementation of the LK Scar Test for the Deep Layers**
>
> To reach and test the deep tissue layers, you need the scoop grip. The exact instructions can be found in Sect. 3.4. A precise setup of this handle is crucial to tension the adhesions well into the depth and to get a clear result. The LK focus here is on the tissue layers **below** the scar in the depth of the tissue.
>
> For an additional provocation or reinforcement, you can further intensify the scoop grip by closing the fingertips even more strongly. Now it is possible to move the fold in different directions. How does the end of these movements feel? Is it elastic and soft and can be easily pushed or pulled? Or is it hard, firm, uncomfortable and feels like a hard stop?

Evaluation

If the end of the movement is soft, elastic, movable and feels inconspicuous, this means that the tissue layers are well movable to each other and there are no adhesions present. The tissue is still movable despite the scoop grip, the grip itself is not particularly uncomfortable. There is no unpleasant pull into the deep tissue layers.

If the scoop grip and the subsequent movement of the layers, however, trigger an end feeling that is hard, firm, inelastic and uncomfortable, then the tissue is glued. A deep pull and tension feeling that extends far into other areas of the body or pulls is a clear sign of this.

The next step is the implementation of an LK treatment e.g. with local techniques for the depth (see Figs. 4.10 and 4.11) or with an LK self-exercise.

3.5.3 Check-in Function/Motion

Normal tissue layers have the ability to move multidimensionally relative to each other. This allows the layers to move or use different parts of the body simultaneously and in opposition to each other. For example, we can dance, raise our arm, turn our head, walk, run or jump, turn around and laugh, digest, breathe, move our joints and cushion movements all at the same time.

As soon as adhesions in the abdominal cavity affect these large movement systems, movements no longer flow smoothly through the entire body, but are unfavorably altered. Compensations in the form of increased muscle tension occur in the body, as the body must combine forces and muscles differently to enable a desired movement pattern. Adhesions create tension lines in the tissue. If you want to move, it may be that it pinches and tweaks at different places and becomes uncomfortable, or you may not be able to bend over at all because the tension in the back does not allow it.

To get into the desired movement, you now use muscle power. In the long run, this constant overloading of the muscles and the extra tension can result in back pain.

Unfortunately, it is often the case that you are not consciously aware of all this, as the healthy tissue around the surgical area is maximally movable and can compensate for the adhesions for a long time. Therefore, we should test certain areas in motion to make hidden restrictions noticeable and visible.

Execution of the LK Scar Function Test

For the test, you grip the area you want to test with the scoop grip. As soon as you have reached a feeling of good tension and notice the end of the movability in the tissue, you add the desired movement impulse that you want to test. For example, you can START moving the hip joint, the spine or the upper body, tilting or turning. But you can also walk through the room, circle the pelvis, go down stairs, move the arm, get up from sitting, circle or tilt the pelvis while sitting, or also turn and twist the upper body... Choose ONE movement and please be mindful and slow in the movement impulses in any case. If adhesions are present, too fast movements can lead to a sudden and intense pain. Basically, it is always about mindfully finding out whether the desired movement can be performed at all and if so, whether the full range of motion (maximally large and maximally far) is possible.

You can test and treat every joint movement and every movement pattern in relation to the scar and the deep adhesions.

The result is again assessed based on the feasibility, the smoothness, the continuity and the end feeling of the tissue. Adhesions are characterized by a much higher pain intensity due to the ingrown pain sensors than normal connective tissue.

An intensification of the test is achieved by mindfully consciously exceeding and overstressing the already reached end of the tissue movability. To do this, continue the movement that you have started to test even further. Even if you feel that the limit has already been reached.

Evaluation

If the end of the movement is soft, elastic, movable and feels inconspicuous, this means that the tissue layers are well movable relative to each other and there are no adhesions present. The tissue is then still movable despite the scoop grip, the grip itself is not particularly uncomfortable. There is no movement restriction or unpleasant pull into the deep tissue layers in the tested movement patterns.

However, if the scoop grip and the subsequent movement impulse trigger an end feeling that is hard, firm, inelastic and uncomfortable, this means that the tissue is adhered. At the same time, a deep pulling and tension feeling often appears, which can reach and pull far into other areas of the body. Any tension that occurs or intensifies uncomfortably is an indicator of impaired movement and sliding systems due to adhesions.

The next step is to perform an LK treatment, for example with the LK self-exercises.

> **Tip**
>
> When you feel only free movement and can test comfortably, the tissue is smooth.
>
> When the movement of the tissue is limited and pulls uncomfortably or is painful at the same time, you have found adhesions. You are exactly right there. Diagnosis: There is only a yes or no.

3.6 The Levels of Scar Treatment

In the treatmentof scars, three levels are distinguished: scar tissue, adhesions in the tissue, and adhesions / growths in the abdominal cavity. All three levels have already been examined in detail in the first part of the guide. How do these three levels feel in practice or in the context of treatment? Depending on the compaction and restriction of movement of the affected person, they are perceived very differently. Therefore, it usually takes different lengths of time for the desired success to be achieved in individual applications.

> **Perceiving Differences**
>
> Scar tissue
>
> - Visible surface: white, reddened, thin, thick, raised, flat, widened-pulled apart

- Tangible feeling: firm, dense and compact, little to no elasticity, burning, stinging, tingling, numb feeling, hypersensitive
- Therapy: slow change in self-treatment, requires a lot of time and frequent applications

Adhesions in the tissue

- Tangible feeling: pulling in the tissue; possible at rest and during movement, dense, lumpy, hardened, firm, flatly compacted under the skin
- Therapy: rapid change in tensile stress during LK self-exercise and decrease of the hard end feeling at the end of movement

Growths inthe abdominal cavity

- Tangible feeling: dense, hard resistance, sometimes felt like "ropes" under the skin, depending on the severity also perceivable as a dense, flat knot in the tissue
- Therapy: depending on the severity, rapid and slow change is possible

In addition, the emotional component should not be forgotten as a fourth level! If the scar is associated with a negative emotional experience or a feeling of danger and fear, this can leave tension in the tissue and reduced tissue mobility. This tension often manifests itself in inhibitions or a complete aversion to dealing with one's own scar, touching or moving it. Some people even suppress the fact that the scar exists.

In these cases, even gentle touches can be experienced as intense and barely bearable. Dealing with the scar and the surgical experience then requires trust and time. It is important to choose the right time to gradually approach the experience again and to give the brain the opportunity to separate the memory from reality, to experience it anew and to re-evaluate it. Once the affected person reaches this moment, major changes and a decrease in tissue tension can quickly occur.

> *"A real change can only occur when the body learns that the danger is over and it is living in the present reality again."* (Van der Kolk 2016, p. 113).

Patient Angela, 34 years old.

> *"It feels so incredibly good not to be at the mercy of back pain. The LK self-exercises are uncomfortable, but at the same time immediate change and relief are noticeable. And with every grip, my scar feels a little softer and my body overall lighter. Also, breathing into the stomach is freer again."*

3.7 Delineation from Other Scar Treatment Concepts

Most methods primarily focus their treatment focus on the visible scar and the superficial tissue layers. Their primary concern is to relax these tissue layers and to dissolve superficially palpable knots.

Compared to the Liedler Concept, the main focus here is on the superficially visible scar and on the reduction of existing inflammatory processes. However, an aspect that I consider important is neglected here: scars that appear to be freely movable on the surface can have adhesions in the deep tissue layers and adhesions in the depth of the abdominal cavity that go unnoticed, but can trigger tension and pain in the rest of the body (Liedler 2017). Unfortunately, there is hardly any literature that describes a concrete influence on adhesions in the tissue, adhesions in the abdominal cavity or the restoration of the sliding layers or the promotion and stimulation of synovial fluids. These aspects are also hardly considered in the various manual therapeutic training centers in the teaching lessons.

What distinguishes the Liedler Concept from other scar treatment concepts in particular? This is easily explained: This special treatment focus achieves a tensioning of the adhesion chains down into the depth. Clear movement impulses, which are specifically aimed at the adhesions (Punktum fixum and Punktum mobile), show restrictions of the sliding layers in the movement system of our body, and make them palpable and treatable. By including extensive movement axes and joint movements in the LK self-exercises, exactly those adhesions are targeted and remodeled that actually cause restrictions in the movement system.

It often shows in practice that physical, painful compensation patterns develop especially when the scar, adhesions in the tissue and adhesions in the abdominal cavity restrict the normal freedom of movement of the surrounding joints and movement axes. So, in normal cases, all joints should always be able to move freely and painlessly in all directions to their maximum extent, regardless of whether adhesions exist or not.

3.8 The Topic of Pain in the Liedler Concept

What effects do pains have on our body? How are pain information perceived and processed? Can pain possibly also be a useful helper during self-treatment and if so, how? This chapter provides information about the definition of pain and sheds light on acute and chronic pain. It is explained in detail what role pain plays in the Liedler Concept and why the Liedler techniques can be uncomfortable or painful. Possible correlations between adhesions in the tissue and adhesions in the abdominal cavity with chronic pain conditions are described as well as the development of protective postures. The focus is on how the Liedler techniques can have a positive influence here.

3.8.1 Pain as Communication of the Body

Pain is fundamentally a warning signal in the body. It points to a possible danger or tissue damage and is supposed to protect us and our body.

However, the actual experience of pain only happens with processing in the brain. The perception and meaning of pain depends on different factors. There are different types of pain, depending on which systems in the body are affected. While own receptors in the tissue determine and assess the position and posture of the body in space, protection against damaging influences is carried out via special nerve cells, the pain receptors. Normally, pain receptors are activated when acting stimuli such as pressure, tension, heat or cold or inflammation-promoting substances exceed a certain intensity and possibly threaten tissue damage. Our nervous system can react to stimuli in seconds. That means, it can quickly filter out damaging stimuli and report tissue injuries and inflammations. In this way, damaging influences can be avoided in the best case and corresponding reactions or adaptations in the body can be carried out.

Even after a surgery, information about our body is constantly transmitted to the brain in relation to the scar, adhesions in the tissue and adhesions in the abdominal cavity, even without conscious pain perception taking place. Unconsciously, movements and behavior can thus arise to protect the tissue and ultimately protective postures.

In the context of the LK, the uncomfortable or painful perception is primarily used as a communication aid to detect the adhesions and their related movement restrictions. Subsequently, the ability of our body to initiate remodeling processes in the tissue through set stimuli is used to change and break down the adhesions. This creates the opportunity on both a conscious and emotional level to re-experience and evaluate the current state of the scar and the associated experiences. New perspectives can be developed that allow changes and deviations in the symptomatology to be registered during the self-exercise and subsequently in everyday life.

3.8.2 Acute Pain

Acute pain is fundamentally linked to a current event or triggering factors. The main symptoms are redness, increased warmth in the affected area, swelling, pain, and loss of function or movement.

Acute pain can last only a few seconds, but also weeks. Every pain is always a warning signal for the body. It is about averting further consequential damage. However, pain can also be errors in the pain signaling system. This is basically designed to avoid damage and pain in advance. Characteristic of acute pain is that it disappears after the cessation of the intense or damaging stimulus or after the end of the triggered inflammation.

In the course of surgeries, acute pain and inflammation are a normal consequence, which can be well controlled with medication. They occur within the first week after the operation and then disappear again.

The symptoms of redness, pain, warmth, and swelling can be observed in a weakened form after the application of the LK self-exercises and indicate successful implementation and the desired tissue remodeling.

3.8.3 Chronic Pain

After major surgery, tissue trauma, nerve injuries, or viral infections, the accompanying inflammatory processes can lead to the development of chronic pain. This means that it persists beyond the duration of normal wound healing processes. Often, chronic pain is associated with a permanent disturbance of tissue structures that is not reversible. Continuous stimuli and tissue overloads then lead to a sensitization of the nervous system as well as to protective postures up to changes in the brain (Gold and Gebhart 2010).

Chronic pain can severely limit quality of life. Common accompanying symptoms are negative moods (up to depression), a change in eating and sleeping behavior (up to insomnia), and generally lacking resources for stress defense (Baliki and Apkarian 2015). This makes chronic pain a complex disease that requires the inclusion of body systems, but also psychological and social levels in the treatment.

Effective therapies for chronic pain are few and far between. The different approaches range from pharmaceutical strategies, nerve stimulation to acupuncture and meditation.

Even after surgery, continuous, chronic pain can occur. If the intervention is far back in the life history, the adhesions in the tissue and adhesions in the abdominal cavity that have arisen are rarely considered as a potential cause, trigger, or contributor to the pain, not specifically included into the treatment. This is where the LK steps in.

Despite long-lasting pain symptoms due to adhesions after abdominal surgeries, existing painful cycles, protective postures, and nerve circuits can be broken and reorganized through their treatment with the LK.

Patient Lore, 57 years after continuous treatments with the Liedler Concept AND regular application of the LK self-exercises:

> *"I never thought that these back pains could still be changed and I never thought that my scars of the surgeries could be related to it. I feel mobile again in my back, that's just great."*

Surgery: Cesarean section 30 years ago, gynecological surgery 10 years ago, appendectomy in adolescence.

Symptoms: chronic back pain for 30 years, sometimes feeling of breaking in the lower back, digestive problems.

3.8.4 Correctly Interpret Pain and Precisely Choose the Intensity of LK Self-Exercises

First and foremost, it should be said that pain is a warning signal of our body and must be respected as such! This means on the one hand, to handle the tolerance limit of pain carefully. On the other hand, it is important to learn to distinguish whether the pain indicates a tissue change or is potentially dangerous. What needs to be considered here? If a discomfort or pain sensation occurs, it is crucial how it behaves subsequently:

Correct interpretation of discomfort or pain and after-reactions when performing the LK self-exercises

- Normal: Uncomfortable strain or an initially short intense, sharp pain that quickly subsides and disappears—complete the exercise!
- Wrong: Appearance of a sharp, burning pain that becomes stronger and feels more threatening during execution—please stop the exercise!

Normal skin reaction after

- Redness
- Slight swelling

> - Slight wound feeling
> - Feeling of muscle soreness

When in doubt, always seek the advice of an expert!

When the stress limit is exceeded, the body will normally react with pain to inform that the stimulus impulses need to be reduced or stopped. We use this information system in the application of LK self-exercises: We "seek" the discomfort (not the pain) to thereby detect adhesions and scar tissue in the body. Subsequently, we use the discomfort during the LK self-exercises, to regulate the intensity to a good measure. Sometimes the initial discomfort is accompanied by stress reactions such as sweating, feeling of heat, tingling, rarely also slight feelings of nausea, dizziness, fog in the head etc. With the progression of the technique, the restoration of the sliding layers and the increase in mobility, these reactions quickly subside. The time of ultimate relaxation always correlates with the noticeable tissue changes and the subsiding of the discomfort. Therefore, it is important for successful application to definitely wait for or reach this moment in order to end in a relaxed body feeling!

> During the LK self-exercises, you have the task and responsibility to accurately adjust your subjectively experienced limits and avoid too intense pain stimuli. The personal **tolerable** pain threshold is **always** in the foreground and must be **lovingly** respected and finely calibrated in combination with the Liedler techniques. A pain perception that leads you to grit your teeth or to let go of the scoop grip due to a sudden shooting pain must definitely be avoided!

If the technique is ended too early, aborted or overdosed, the body remains in an activated stress state, which can lead to unpleasant after-reactions such as discomfort, inner restlessness, a worsening of the experienced body symptoms or also a sensitization of the affected area. Therefore, a precise and loving handling of the LK techniques in self-application is absolutely necessary! If the techniques are nevertheless interrupted, the tissue can be immediately locally calmed and thus unpleasant after-reactions can be intercepted by another precise, loving and **to the end** performed technique. It is important for the maximum success of the self-exercise that the user always experiences a good completion and a relaxed body feeling after each technique!

In the context of LK treatment of adhesions and scar tissue in the abdominal area, often an acute pain occurs initially for a short time. Since the subjectively perceived pain can be co-regulated via the brain (Baliki and Apkarian 2015), it is particularly important to understand the background of the treatment and the reason for the pain during scar therapy. A good and conscious understanding, but also the controllability of the pain event, contribute to the fact that you can perform the LK self-exercises relaxed and efficiently. It is important to know that with the correct execution of the technique, the acute initial discomfort only lasts for a short time and a sharp pain is to be avoided. During the application of the LK self-exercises, there is immediately a noticeable tissue remodeling of the adhesions and the restoration of the sliding layers—this means that the cause of the discomfort or pain (rigid adhesions with ingrown nerve endings instead of flexible tissue structure) and thus also the pain experience disappears. The reason for this lies, among other things, in the fact that the original freedom of movement in the affected area is restored as much as possible. This eliminates the causative continuous irritation. Thus, based on a real tissue change, a new subjective perception and a new body feeling can also arise.

> Choosing a **tolerable** intensity **and** a mindful, precise and loving execution of the LK self-exercise to the end leads to the most mobility, the best relaxation of the body and the greatest success!

3.9 How the Timing of the Operation Affects Therapy

After each surgery, there are different wound healing phases. What does this mean for the application of the Liedler techniques? To answer this question, the treatment options within the individual phases are explained in detail in this chapter. Depending on how long ago the operation was, the application of certain techniques and exercises is recommended or to be avoided for young or old scars.

3.9.1 Accompanying Scars in the Healing Process

During the initial acute phase of wound healing, it is important to protect the scar and the involved tissue layers to ensure that the initial adhesion of the wound can proceed well and efficiently. For the subsequent healing phases, there are different focuses. Gradually, the tissue is rebuilt and functionally aligned accordingly. This means that the movement and everyday stresses to which the body is exposed determine the mobility of the tissue. While initially the aim is to support the body's suppleness through normal everyday movements and sleeping positions, over time, direct and specific LK self-exercises and LK techniques can be applied for support.

3.9.1.1 Young Scars—Day 1 to 5 of Wound Healing

In the first five days of wound healing after surgery, blood clotting, the formation of the first temporary replacement tissue, and the stabilization of the wound occur. During this time, therapies and exercises are only permitted within the **pain-free** range of motion. And this is only under the condition that the affected person has an **adequate pain perception** that is not diminished by the intake of painkillers. Large pressure, tensile, or displacement loads on the fresh scar should be avoided to achieve good closure of the wound and the superficial skin and tissue layers. Powerful and direct techniques or large loads such as muscle training, carrying heavy objects are prohibited in this first phase of wound healing, as they can increase the inflammatory processes and delay wound healing. Deep abdominal breathing is recommended.

3.9.1.2 Young Scars—Day 5 to 10 of Wound Healing

In the following building phase of the tissue from day five, there is a gradual deposition of tissue components and a strengthening of the tissue. To restore and align the tissue structures and their function as originally as possible, it is now important to progressively confront the affected tissue with normal, physiological stress stimuli. It is important to respect one's own pain perception in any case. A loving approach to the body supports a relaxed healing process.

In this phase, you can therefore try and perform individual movement exercises to reduce and dissolve protective postures of the body. Protective postures that usually occur in the first few days, such as avoiding the straightening of the body after abdominal surgery, can thus be consciously counteracted. Test the current range of motion of the joints adjacent to the surgical area and lovingly expand it if necessary. Through deep abdominal breathing, you trigger continuous, gentle movements of the deep abdominal area and the deep sliding layers of the tissue, which support the supply and the swelling of the wound there.

The goal is to set gentle impulses through versatile, different, large-scale movements that correspond to the normal stresses of the body. By moving and using the body as normally as possible, the tissue sliding layers are promoted and supported.

3.9.1.3 Young Scars—Day 10 to 21 of Wound Healing

Around day 10, the layers of the abdominal cavity are already healed. Most patients can usually manage their daily routine quite well again. However, the skin layers and the superficially visible scar still need time to become well established. The formation of new tissue peaks between the sixth and 16th day of wound healing and continues for several more weeks. During this time, the mechanical stress capacity of the scar and its tear resistance also increase (Asmussen and Söllner 2010). This results in the initially noticeable severe movement restrictions usually having significantly decreased by the second and third week after the operation. Movement restrictions and pain are primarily determined by the size and progress of the healing of the skin scar in this context.

However, lifting heavy objects and any intensive strain on the abdominal wall should still be avoided due to the lack of tissue strength of the scar, in order to prevent complications such as scar hernias. It is important that you can assess yourself well, in order to choose the intensity of stresses depending on your own pain experience carefully and specifically.

Occurring complications, open wound sites, and infections can delay the wound healing processes. The affected scar area must then under no circumstances be treated specifically and directly.

In this phase, the main focus of the LK self-applications is on preventing further solidifications of adhesions through **pain-free** and gentle movements. At the same time, the promotion of the sliding layers is now being started.

The superficial scar is included directly or only indirectly depending on its wound closure. The aim is to locally reduce possible tensions in the deeper tissue layers, to maintain or promote the normal sliding properties of the tissue layers, and thus to reduce or dissolve existing protective postures and compensations of the tissue.

3.9.1.4 Scars from the 21st Day of Wound Healing

From day 21, the repair phase nowfollows, which lasts up to a year. During this time, the tissue continues to strengthen and adapt to external influences.

In the LK self-applications, the strain on the tissue is now slowly and steadily increased to drive the remodeling of the tissue according to the physical stresses forward. The intensity should always be based on a well-tolerable subjective pain experience (Van den Berg 2014). **When in doubt, always dose lower!** If your pain and body perception has not yet been well restored or is still impaired by painkillers, direct LK self-exercises should not be started.

As soon as the body can be fully loaded again after the surgery and sports can also be practiced, there is nothing to prevent an LK self-application.

3.9.2 Old Scars

Adhesions in the tissue and in the abdominal cavity vary greatly after surgeries. The more surgeries that have occurred in a person's life and the more time that has passed, the more compensations occur more or less noticeably in the body. Corresponding protective postures, which then persist for a longer period of time, lead to further restructuring and can trigger major changes in the dynamics of the pelvis and back (Heymann and Stecco 2016; Langevin et al. 2011).

Even with old scars, intensive manual pressure and tension impulses in the tissue can stimulate and trigger new remodeling processes.

With old scars, more frequent or comprehensive treatments with the LK may be necessary over a longer period of time to influence the complex interplay of the individual tissue components of the adhesions in the tissue and in the abdominal cavity. Now, the superficial and deep tissue components of the scar should be included in the LK exercises through as many joints and movements as possible. This not only causes a direct tissue remodeling, but also frees the entire associated movement chains and body systems.

Old Scars: Patient M., 62 years old.
Surgery: Cesarean section at 32 years old.
Symptoms: Chronic back pain that was always slightly noticeable; Massages provided temporary relief; occasional shortness of breath.
Course of treatment: The patient came for treatment at regular intervals of three to four weeks over a period of one year. At the same time, she worked regularly and intensively at home with her scar. Even during the time of the first appointments, the appearance of the scar improved. The direct local techniques on the scar, which the patient immediately

implemented herself, supported the fact that the redness and the overhanging tissue fold disappeared within the first 3 months. The pain symptoms also changed noticeably. The patient was able to further reduce her hip pain by applying the LK **toilet dance exercise** and the **stairs exercise**. The constant pain became a fluctuating pain, whose intensity decreased and then occasionally increased again. Pain-free periods began to occur and superficial and deep layers of the scar as well as the mobility of the pelvis and body steadily increased. The breathing deepened. After one year, the chronic back pain, which had already existed for 30 years, finally disappeared completely and the patient was again mobile in the body and pain-free.

References

Asmussen, Peter D., Brigitte Söllner. 2010. Die Prinzipien der Wundheilung. Bd. Sonderausgabe. Embrach:Kammerlander.

Bordoni, Bruno, Escher A.R., Girgenti G.T., Tobbi F., Bonanzinga R. Osteopathic Approach for Keloids and Hypertrophic Scars. Cureus. 2023 Sep 7;15(9):e44815. https://doi.org/10.7759/cureus.44815. PMID: 37692181; PMCID: PMC10483258.

Baliki, M. N, A. V. Apkarian. 2015. „Nociception, Pain, Negative Moods, and Behavior Selection". Neuron 87 (3): 474–91.

Dodd, John G., Meadow Maze Good, Tammy L. Nguyen, Anderson I. Grigg et al. 2006. „In Vitro Biophysical Strain Model for Understanding Mechanisms of Osteopathic Manipulative Treatment". The Journal of the American Osteopathic Association 106 (3): 157–66.

Fourie, W. J. 2014. „Operationen und Narbenbildung". *Lehrbuch Faszien*, herausgegeben von R. Schleip, T. W. Findely, L. Chaitow, P. A. Huijing, 1. Auflage, 308–15. München: Elsevier GmbH.

Gold, M. S., G. F. Gebhart. 2010. „Nociceptor sensitization in pain pathogenesis". Nature medicine 16 (11): 1.248–57.P. A. Huijing, 1. Auflage, 308–15. München: Elsevier GmbH.

Heymann, Wolfgang von, Carla Stecco. 2016. „Fasziale Dysfunktionen". Manuelle Medizin 54: 303–6. https://doi.org/10.1007/s00337-016-0172-1.

Langevin H.M., J. R. Fox, C. Koptiuch, G. J. Badger et al. 2011. „Reduced thoracolumbar fascia shear strain in human chronic low back pain". BMC Musculoskeltal Disorders 12 (203): 1–11.

Liedler, Michaela 2017. „Einfluss von postoperativen Adhäsionen nach Sektio auf chronischen Low Back Pain — eine Pilotstudie". Masterthese, Krems: DUK.

Liedler, Michaela. 2020. „Peritoneale Adhäsionen—Fasziale Behandlung nach dem Liedler-Konzept". Berlin, Heidelberg: Springer Verlag GmbH.

Levin, S. M. 2014. „Biotensegrität-die Faszienmechanik". Lehrbuch Faszien, herausgegeben von R. Schleip, T. W. Findely, L. Chaitow, P. A. Huijing, 1. Auflage, 101–5. München: Urban & Fischer.

Moyer, C.A., J. Rounds, und J.W. Hannum. 2004. „A Meta-Analysis of Massage Therapy Research". Psychological Bulletin 130 (1): 3–18. https://doi.org/10.1037/0033-2909.130.1.3.

Van den Berg, F. 2014. „Die Physiologie der Faszie". Lehrbuch Faszien, herausgegeben von R. Schleip, T. W. Findely, L. Chaitow, P. A. Huijing, 1. Auflage, 110–14. München: Elsevier GmbH.

Van der Kolk, B.A. 2015. Verkörperter Schrecken: Traumaspuren in Gehirn, Geist und Körper und wie man sie heilen kann. Lichtenau: G. B. Probst Verlag.

4

Practice—HandsOn

In the operating room, every patient loses their autonomy at the start of the surgery. Trusting that the doctor will act in their best interest, the patient must essentially "surrender" to the situation. This feeling of powerlessness is felt more strongly by some than others. The clear and effective agency of the active self-exercises of the Liedler Concept not only counteracts the effects of scars and adhesions, but also this feeling of powerlessness: a new access to one's own body **with** a scar is created. At the same time, you can proactively treat potential negative effects of the surgery and thereby reduce chronic pain. A sense of well-being, deep breathing, and lightness return to the body.

4.1 Practical Recommendations and Self-Exercises

4.1.1 Dealing with Young Scars

This chapter provides valuable practical advice so that you can support yourself well during the first few days after the surgery. Practical recommendations and self-exercises are explained for young scars to support wound

---

Supplementary Information The online version contains supplementary material available at https://doi.org/10.1007/978-3-662-71377-8_4. The videos can be accessed individually by clicking the DOI link in the accompanying figure caption or by scanning this link with the SN More Media App.

healing and swelling reduction, maintain tissue suppleness, and prevent or counteract the formation of adhesions in the abdominal area.

4.1.1.1 First Week

In the first week (see Fig. 4.1) after the surgery, the focus is primarily on dealing with the changes in the body and positively encountering the appearance and new feeling of skin and tissue. The following movement instructions are derived from normal everyday life. With them, we support the reduction of swelling, the supply of tissue, and the glideability of the layers in the abdominal area during the first wound healing phase.

- Gentle touching and creaming, as soon as the plaster is removed, help to get in touch with the scar.
- Conscious deep breathing into the abdomen and pelvic area—ideally 24 hours a day, 7 days a week—gently and steadily supports tissue supply and swelling reduction.
- Different lying and sleeping positions—as soon as they are possible and comfortably bearable—help the sliding layers to stay in motion where the body needs it, to take positions relaxedly and to prevent adhesions in these areas.

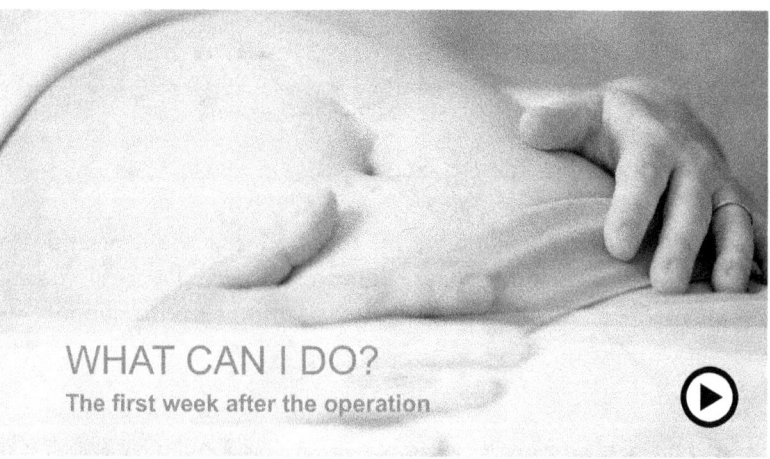

Fig. 4.1 The first week after the surgery. (@ 2023 Liedler-Concept. What am I allowed to do? The first week after the operation ▸ https://doi.org/10.1007/000-fs6)

- After abdominal surgery, sitting up in bed and getting up should still be done via the side to relieve the scar and keep the direct tension in the affected area low.
- Protective postures should be consciously but still cautiously reduced. This means that slowly you can start with normal straightening and moving of the body as well as with mindful walks.

4.1.1.1.1 First Haptic Approach (Touching, Creaming)

Since a surgery represents a real incision, this is about actual changes in the body. The skin and tissue feel different and also behave unusually in movement. The rest of the body is primarily challenged by pain and corresponding protective postures in the initial stage. In this phase, looking at the scar helps us understand how and what is now different than before. A first touch and creaming help to get to know the **new** and **unknown**. It is important to "grasp" with the fingers how the scar, the skin, and possible tissue changes now feel. Many initially experience a feeling of discomfort or disgust. If this is the case, it is advisable to first feel different qualities at other parts of the body: A bone feels hard and sometimes also edgy, tendons round and firm, tissue on the stomach normally soft and elastic, muscles can offer different sensory qualities from soft to firm. As varied as our body feels, so varied are the scars. They are usually very firm and inelastic, but not necessarily. Under the skin, it is also possible to feel other lumps and firmer spots, sometimes also strands and cords. These are then adhesions in the underlying tissue. Do you sense and discover differences? Recognizing that there is other unfamiliarity to experience in and on the body besides the scar often makes it easier to deal with the scar by touch.

4.1.1.1.2 Abdominal Breathing

Relaxed and correct abdominal breathing (see Figs. 4.2, 4.3 and 4.4) supports the reduction of swelling, the supply of tissue, and the healing processes. The breath gently oscillates through the body—the large breathing muscle (the diaphragm), in conjunction with the pelvic floor, gently rocks and keeps the entire abdominal area in motion. Deep abdominal breathing activates the nervous system responsible for relaxation and regeneration processes in the body. With the support of good breathing, the body can not only more easily reduce tension, but the state of relaxation is also activated.

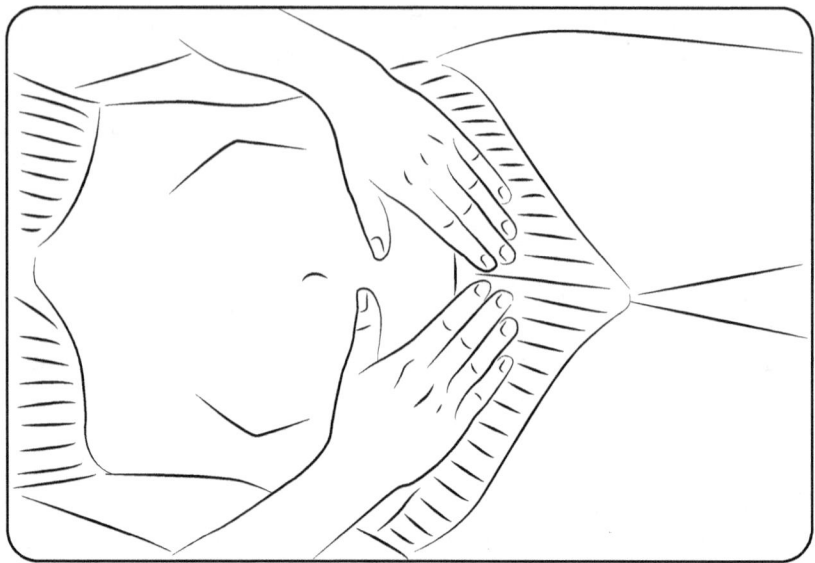

Fig. 4.2 Abdominal breathing—with hands on the lower abdomen

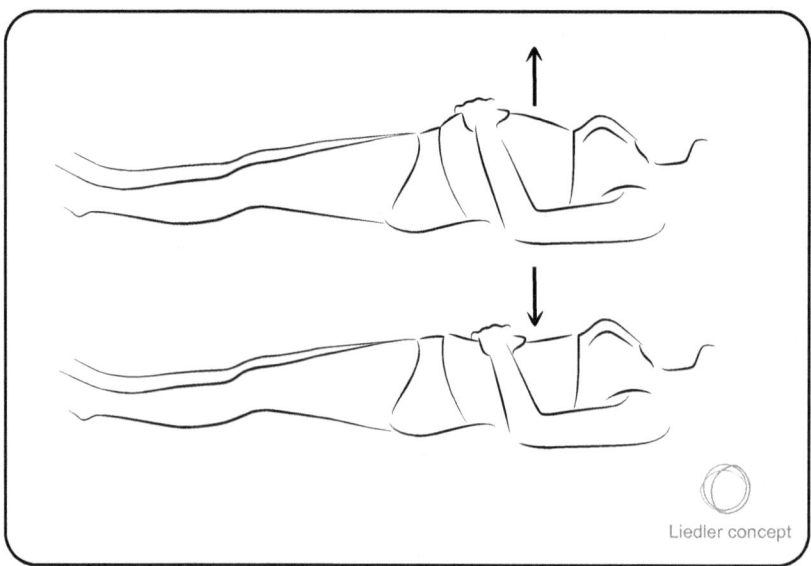

Fig. 4.3 Abdominal breathing—Inhalation and exhalation. (@ 2023 Liedler-Concept)

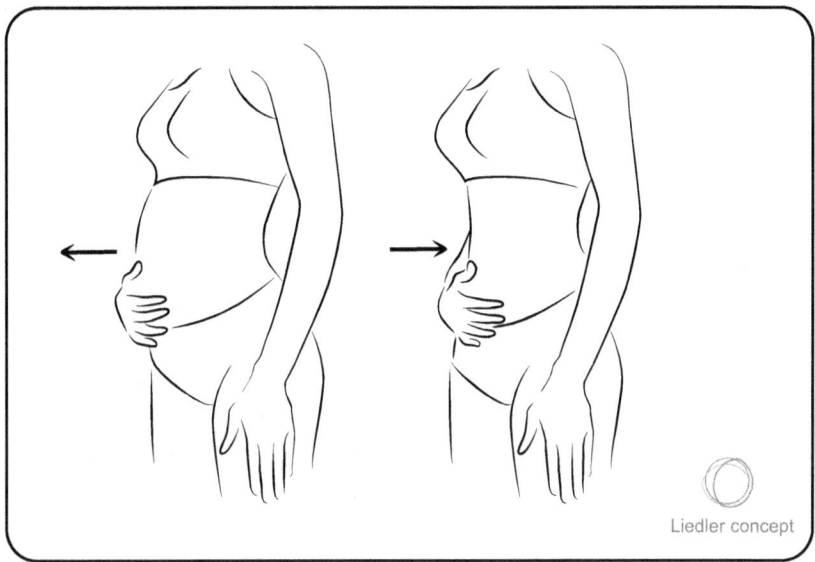

Fig. 4.4 Abdominal breathing—Inhalation and exhalation standing. (@ 2023 Liedler-Concept)

You can tell this specifically by the fact that the pulse slows down and blood pressure drops. Often the stomach starts to gurgle and rumble—this is also a sign of relaxation.

Execution of abdominal breathing

- The simplest starting position to learn abdominal breathing is the supine position. Either place both hands lovingly on your lower abdomen or one hand on the lower abdomen and the second under your back. Direct the breath deep into the pelvis. When inhaling, you should now feel how the abdominal wall lifts with your hands and at the same time extends towards the base into the back. When exhaling, the stomach sinks in and the navel can be gently pulled inward towards the spine. The breath should flow gently.
- If that works well, try the breathing while sitting. Again, place your hands on the lower abdomen. The stomach may now "fall between the legs" when inhaling. At the same time, the breath may also expand into the lower back. When exhaling, the stomach is pulled back towards the spine over the navel. The abdominal muscles thus gently help to push the air back up.

- The next increase is to test the breathing in an upright position. Here too, it is helpful for the body if you place your hands on the lower abdomen and on the lower back.
- In general, it would be great if you could maintain this form of breathing during any movement and make deep abdominal breathing a part of your everyday life.

Incorrect: Often it happens that the chest is raised and the stomach is drawn in when inhaling. When exhaling, the stomach is then pushed down and out with pressure. This simultaneously increases the intra-abdominal pressure and pushes the wound apart. The result is often that you stop breathing into the stomach altogether because of the uncomfortable feeling.

The goal is for this abdominal breathing to always be and remain part of the breathing, 24 hours a day, 7 days a week. Regardless of the position and situation and active activity. But beware, it takes many repetitions until this happens automatically. Be patient with yourself here, it's worth it. The body is automatically balanced into a more relaxed basic state through the correct deep abdominal breathing.

4.1.1.1.3 Sleeping—How Should I Lie?

The first tissue connections form during wound healing within hours after surgery. Therefore, it makes sense to change positions frequently early on to prevent adhesions and support the sliding and flexibility of the tissue layers. This way, we can also prevent tension caused by one-sided positions and postures. This is particularly relevant for sleeping, as we remain in the same position for hours, often due to pain, but also out of fear that another position could cause damage. Try lying and sleeping in different positions over time to see if the side position, the half-side position, or the prone position are also comfortable and relieving. It is usually very relieving for the rest of your body if you bring variety into your positioning.

However, it should be noted that it is NEVER about changing to painful positions, let alone staying in them! A new position may initially feel uncomfortable or trigger a pulling sensation in the tissue. But this should always quickly subside and turn into a relaxed feeling. Any pain, triggered by a new movement or position, that progressively worsens instead of subsiding, should ALWAYS be immediately resolved!

4.1.1.1.4 Moving in Everyday Life

Due to the pain in the first few days after surgery, conscious and unnoticed protective postures usually develop. To prevent these from becoming a habit and changing the body in the long term, you should become aware of your protective postures on the one hand and, on the other hand, resort to them as briefly as possible and dissolve them as soon as possible, adapted to the pain.

The following list of the most common protective postures is intended to help recognize them as such.

> **Common protective postures**
> - Shallow, superficial breathing, especially into the chest
> - Stooped posture
> - Bent back
> - Forward shoulders
> - Lack of upper body straightening
> - Small steps when walking
> - Uncertain steps when walking
> - Avoidance of rotational movements of the upper body or the affected area
> - Avoidance of certain movements, not utilizing the maximum possible range of motion
> - Avoidance of certain sleep positions, such as prone position, side position, half-side position, or supine position
> - Persistently increased tension in the body or in certain parts of the body—stiff feeling

Generally, the aim is for you to move and behave as normally as possible during this phase, just as the pain and uncomfortable feeling allow. The goal is for you to return to your normal everyday movements and range of motion as soon as possible and not to develop additional adhesions and restrictions in the tissue based on the protective postures.

4.1.1.2 Second Week to Sixth Week

Starting from the second week, you can actively contribute to the new tissue being built as flexible, dynamic, and resilient as possible. The following recommendations will help.

- As in the first week, continue to focus on deep and conscious breathing. The exercise "belly breathing pump" (see below Sect. 4.1.1.2.2) can further enhance this effect.
- Change your sleeping positions: supine, prone, lateral, and semi-prone.
- Start with mindful body exercises to counteract protective postures: alternating leg extensions in supine position, gentle chest stretching, rotational movements of the thoracic spine while sitting, gentle stretching and alternating arm extensions over the head (like "picking apples"), slow descending and ascending, measured stair climbing.
- Gentle scar mobilization can now also be started.
- From the third week onwards, a continuous, individually adapted increase in everyday movements is recommended—after consultation with the surgeon. This also includes asking when you can resume your sexual life, as this moves, promotes, and keeps the deep layers in the pelvis flexible maintained.

4.1.1.2.1 Abdominal Breathing

The exercises for abdominal breathing were written in detail in Sect. 4.1.1.2.2 Abdominal Breathing.

4.1.1.2.2 Variant: Abdominal-Air-Pump

With the help of the so-called "belly breathing pump", the displacement effect of tissue glide layers and organs can be further enhanced. The production of lubricating fluids in the tissue and in the abdominal cavity is also more strongly stimulated by this.

> **Instructions for the Deep Belly Breathing Pump**
>
> For this exercise, it is a prerequisite that you are already very proficient in the technique of deep abdominal breathing. For the belly breathing pump, breathe in moderately deep and then hold your breath for the entire exercise. If necessary, you can also close your nose with two fingers. Now try to "inhale" air through the closed nose. This will automatically push the abdomen out. Then try to "exhale". This pulls the navel towards the spine and slightly activates the abdominal muscles through active mindful retraction of the abdomen. Repeat the cycle of "inhaling and exhaling" 3 to 5 times, then pause and repeat it twice more. The pressure shifts and the movement that is transmitted to the abdominal cavity via the respiratory muscles and the pelvic floor ensure a displacement of tissue, organs, and fluids. This supports both the movement and the flexibility in the abdominal cavity.

4.1.1.2.3 *Moving the Scar: Shifting, Lifting*

Once the crust has detached and the scar becomes visible, it can be assumed that the wound is well closed. At this point, the scar usually feels very firm and inelastic. In places, redness, numb or hypersensitive areas may occur, caused by tissue damage or nerves grown into adhesions. The rigid and firm tissue structures of the scar can cause persistent irritation. The sooner the tissue in this area becomes soft and flexible again, the faster the skin's sensation normalizes and redness decreases.

When moving the scar (see Fig. 4.5), it is important to always approach it with mindfulness, as the firmness of the scar only reaches its maximum strength after weeks and months. This also means that the edges of the scar should NEVER be pulled apart when moving and mobilizing!

- To gently mobilize the scar, make contact with the skin: with the fingertips on one side of the scar, with the thumbs on the other side. The scar is now in the middle between thumb and fingers. Now try to move the scar as a whole back and forth, without sliding your fingers over the skin. You can also gently move the scar against each other with your hands like a snake. Initially, you usually feel hard movement limits in the tissue instead of a soft shiftability. The longer you continue the same movement

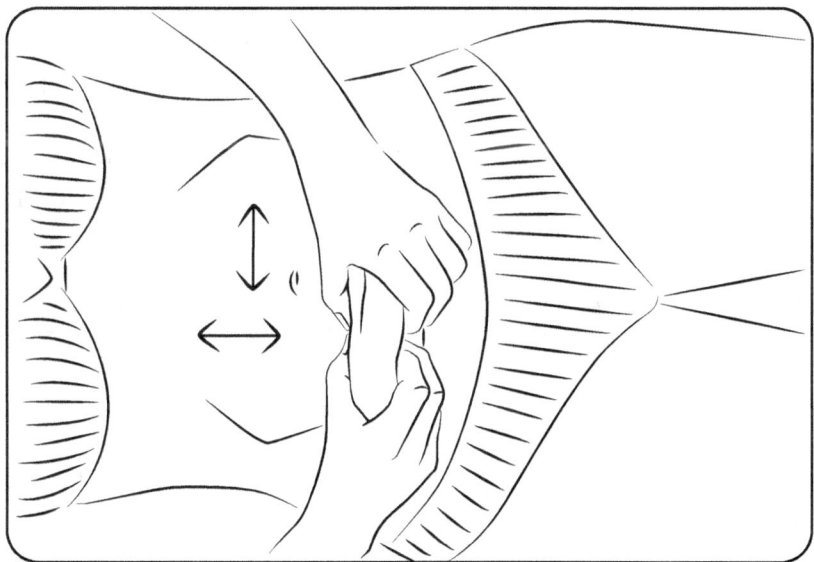

Fig. 4.5 Moving the Scar

(not several different directions at once!), the softer the tissue should feel and the initially unpleasant feeling should subside.
- You can now also try to lift the scar slightly. It is advisable to only grasp and lift small areas for larger scars. Lifting the entire scar is usually not possible due to the underlying adhesions.
- Nodules or lumps that you may feel under the skin surface can be massaged with circular movements. Normally, this initially feels uncomfortable or painful, but relaxes during the massaging movement.

The goal is for the scar and the top, adjacent tissue layers to become supple and soft again.

4.1.1.2.4 Moving the Rest of the Body—Everyday Movements, Stretching of the body

Everyday movements can now gradually be expanded by different larger movements to counteract protective postures and extend the range of motion.

I recommend the following movements (see Figs. 4.6, 4.7, 4.8 and 4.9), which should be mindfully repeated until the movement feels pleasant and smooth:

- **Lengthening the legs:** You lie on your back and alternately lengthen your legs, once to the left, once to the right. For this, you push the entire extended leg towards the foot. This correctly shifts the pelvis alternately towards the feet.
- **Lengthening the arms:** In a supine position, sitting or standing, you stretch your arms far above your head. As if you wanted to "pick apples" alternately with your arms, you now reach far up with your arm, alternately left and right.
- **Lengthening the arms and legs together:** In a supine position, these two exercises can be combined very well. For this, you first lengthen the entire left side and then the entire right side. You mindfully alternate this large and long movement a few times and observe whether the range of motion increases and the smoothness improves. As an increase, you can now try whether you can also maximally lengthen diagonally: this means that you now stretch the left arm and at the same time lengthen the right leg towards the foot. And then combine the right arm with the left leg.

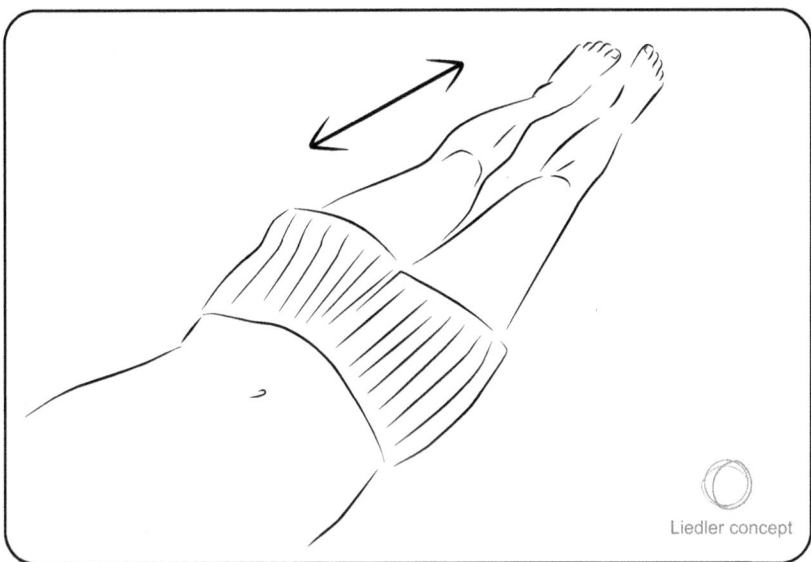

Fig. 4.6 Lengthening the legs. (@ 2023 Liedler-Concept)

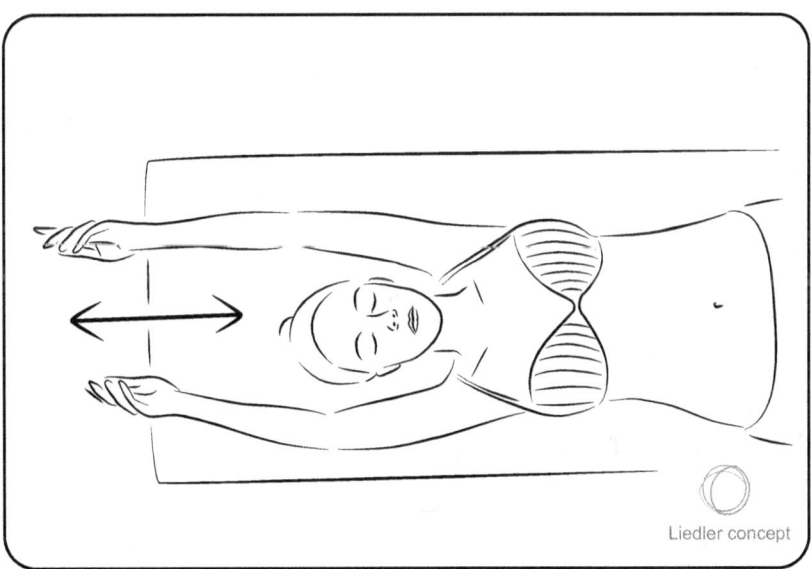

Fig. 4.7 Lengthening the arms. (@ 2023 Liedler-Concept)

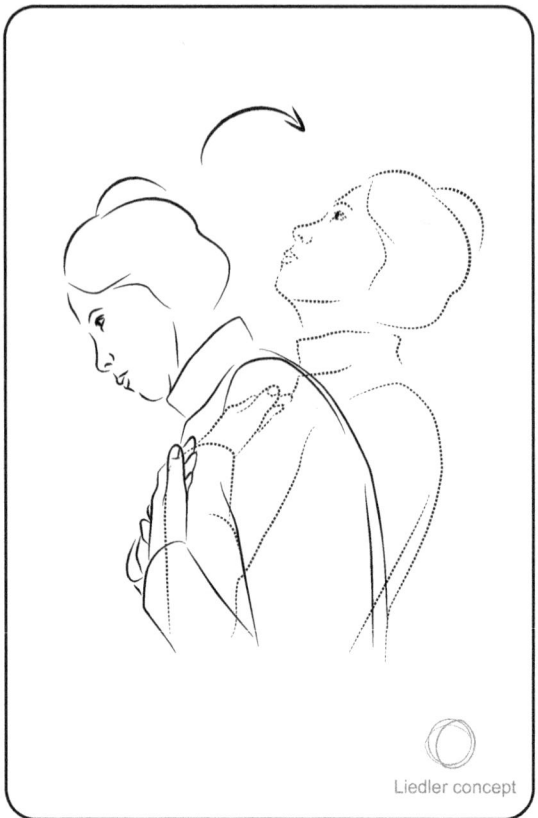

Fig. 4.8 Opening the chest. (@ 2023 Liedler-Concept)

- **Opening the chest:** In a supine position, sitting or standing, you place one hand on your sternum in the middle of the chest. Then try to push your hand forward and up from the part of the thoracic spine between the shoulder blades that is opposite your hand. The shoulders remain relaxed. Go back to the initial position and repeat a couple of times.
- **Rotating the upper body:** Try to sit up as straight as possible and then rotate the upper body as far as possible to the left and then as far as possible to the right. Repeat these movements mindfully a few times. The head can be rotated with the chest or kept straight in the middle, so that only the chest is twisted.
- **Walking downhill, going down stairs:** When you go down stairs or walk downhill in open terrain, make sure that your upper body remains as upright as possible. You may feel a pulling sensation in the scar area or the front area of the body. These are the adhesions that make it difficult for

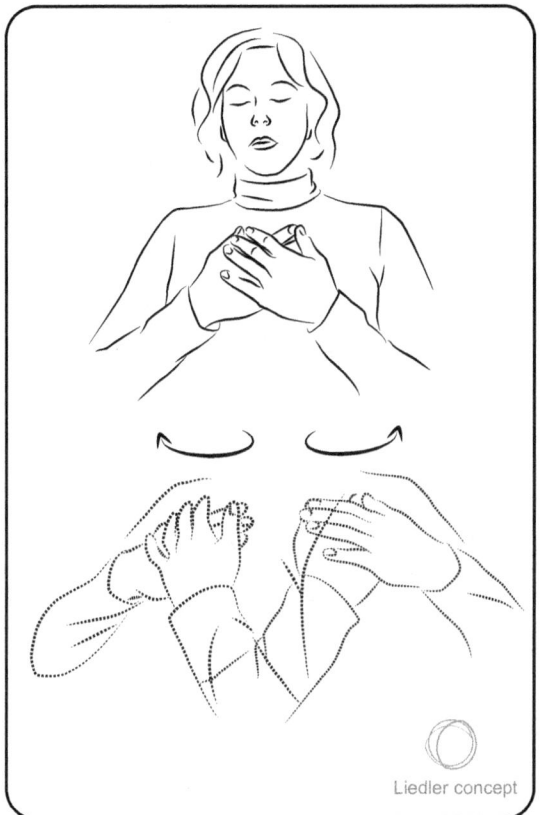

Fig. 4.9 Rotating the upper body. (@ 2023 Liedler-Concept)

you to lengthen and shift the layers of tissue at this moment. Always stay mindful and attentive and continue until the pull decreases significantly, by at least two thirds, and you feel smoother and lighter.

4.1.1.2.5 Sleeping—How Should I Lie?

You can find the recommendations for sleeping positions in Sect. 4.1.1.3.

4.1.1.3 Dealing with Scars from Week 7

As soon as the surgeon gives the clearance for normal loads and also sports activities, you can start working directly with the adhesions in the tissue and in the abdominal cavity. Normally, this is about the seventh week after the operation. Depending on your own individual professional and sporting demands on your own body, treatment should now be carried out directly where the restrictions are specifically found, in order to restore the best possible original state.

The older the scar and the more surgeries have taken place in the life history, the more areas and affected layers of the body will need to be treated. Frequent and regular application of the LK self-exercises over a longer period of time may be necessary to achieve the desired success. However, it is always the case that every effectively treated, newly movable and free tissue guide layer is automatically integrated into the body's movement axes and adopted. Protective postures in the tissue are therefore no longer necessary and the released and movable layers all remain.

> If you get the feeling that no improvement is occurring, please check your scoop grip, the LK focus, and the exact structure and sequence of the exercise. Please remember that there are many layers of tissue in the body that want to become mobile again in many directions of movement! If in doubt, consult an LK expert!

The treatment according to the Liedler Concept includes the following levels:

- Moving the scar (with closed wound)
- The treatment of adhesions in the abdominal cavity in the superficial and deep tissue layers using Local Technique (LT) and LK self-exercises (toilet dance exercise, stairs exercise, individually adapted LK exercises)
- The inclusion of abdominal breathing and its application in everyday life (24 h/7 days a week)

4.1.1.3.1 Local Techniques

To make the tissue layers adjacent to the scar locally supple, the local techniques of the Liedler Concept (LT 1, LT 2) are suitable (see Fig. 4.10).

> **Instructions for Local Technique 1**
> With the first local LK-Technique (LT 1), small and dense areas can be treated well. For the LT 1, the scar is grasped with both hands using the scoop grip. Make sure that both the fingers among each other and the index fingers and

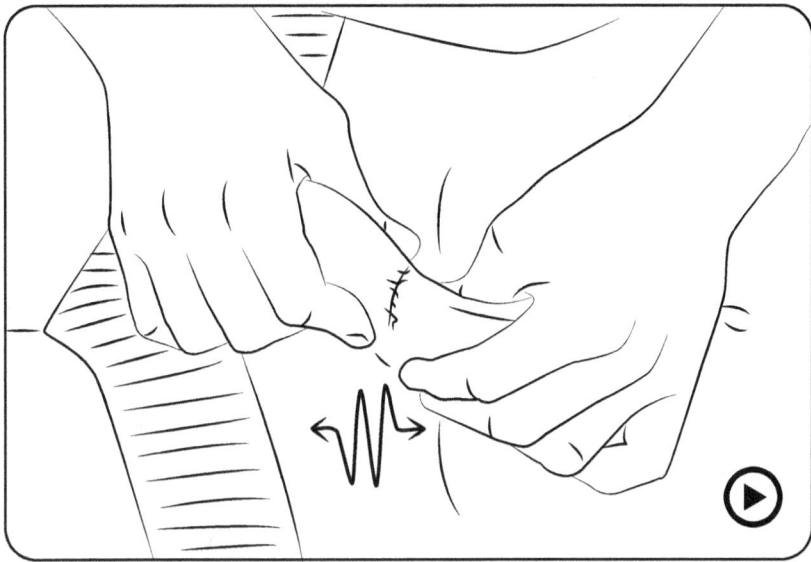

Fig. 4.10 Local Technique 1. (©2023 Liedler Concept ▸ https://doi.org/10.1007/000-fs5)

thumbs of both hands touch each other. The fold between the fingers can be as large as possible. The smaller the fold, the more difficult it is to fix the adhesions. Please remember that the adhesions between tissue layers under the skin correspond to the iceberg. We now want to break this iceberg into individual small puzzle pieces. For this, we focus with both hands on a small area of about 1 cm^2 below the scar in the depth of the layers.

Once both hands have firmly grasped the scar with the scoop grip, one hand now remains still (Punktum fixum), while the other hand (Punktum mobile) performs small, mindful, dynamic pendulum movements over the tissue boundary and back to it.

The end of the technique is reached when the movement is easy to perform, the tissue feels elastic and soft again, and the intensity or pulling has decreased by at least two thirds compared to the beginning.

Important

It is important here that the LK focus (see Sect. 3.3) always lies in the depth below the scar. Since the maximum strength of the scar is only reached after weeks or months, this also avoids deliberately pulling apart the edges of the scar!

The thumb and fingers always enclose the scar from both sides, so that the scar practically lies tension-free in the middle. The LK focus is in the depth below the scar. The moment the adjacent tissue layers in the depth of the scar become movable, there is automatically less tension on the scar, and it can subsequently be integrated more softly and better into the area.

Guide Local Technique 2

The second local LK-Technique of the Liedler Concept (LT 2) (see Fig. 4.11) is suitable for large compacted and adhered areas around and below the scar. These areas can often be recognized by the fact that the tissue slips away under the fingers and cannot be held well.

For the LT 2, **one** puzzle piece of the iceberg is encompassed with both hands with the scoop grip (Punctum fixum form the fixed adhesions). In contrast to the LT 1, the tissue is now simultaneously moved, distorted, and moved back and forth across the tissue boundary with both hands (Punctum mobile).

The end is also reached here when the felt resistance under the skin and the pulling or uncomfortable feeling has decreased by at least two-thirds compared to the beginning and the tissue can be moved softly again.

The targeted and tangible changes always describe how sliding layers are freed, loosened, and how the adhesions change. This way, you can directly experience and learn how immobility becomes mobility and flexible tissue again.

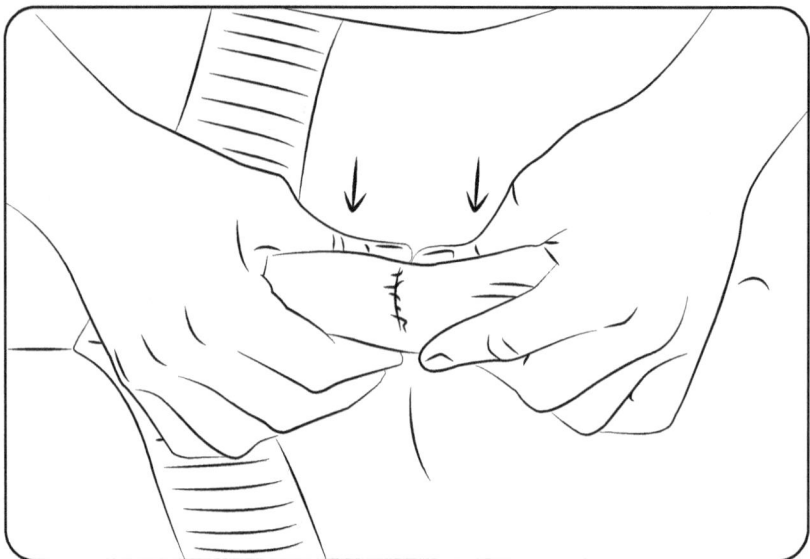

Fig. 4.11 Local Technique 2

4.1.1.3.2 *NART - Movement Exercise*

The direct movement approach of LK self-exercises is suitable for specifically restricted directions of movement and movement patterns in the body. This connection of the **S**car with actual movements of the surrounding joints (medically: **ART**iculation) is also referred to as NART technique in the Liedler Concept. The toilet dance exercise is particularly suitable for the abdominal area (see Figs. 4.12, 4.13 and 4.14), in which the scar is directly related to the movement restrictions and is simultaneously freed. Simple, immediately noticeable, really effective and sustainable.

> **Toilet Dance Exercise Instructions**
>
> The exercise always begins in a sitting position. Why? When sitting, the abdomen is relaxed and the adhesions can be easily grasped. With both hands, a part of the scar is encompassed with the scoop grip and fixed together with the affected tissue layers in depth. With the correct scoop grip, an unpleasant to painful tension should now be noticeable in the targeted tissue. This tension is now held fixed (Punktum fixum). In the next step, you slowly and carefully stand up. Slowly is important because you do not yet know when the adhesions will really start to pull and possibly cause pain. You may not be able to stand up straight away.

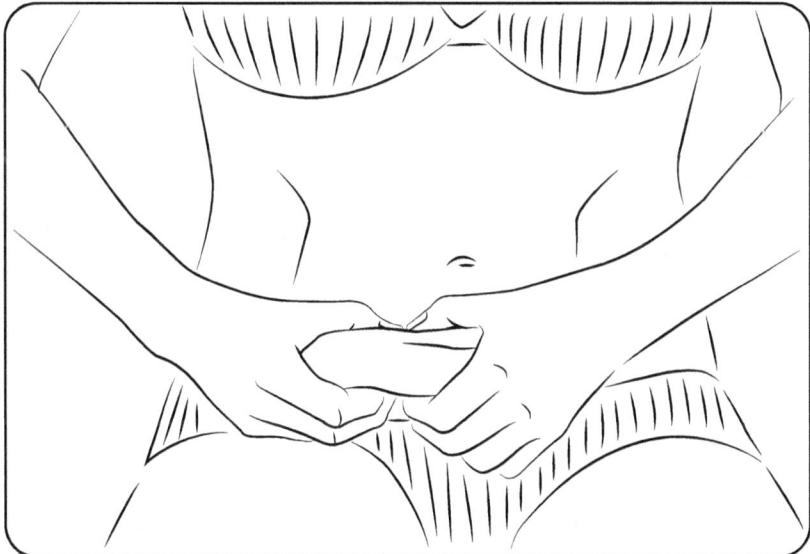

Fig. 4.12 Toilet dance exercise hand position

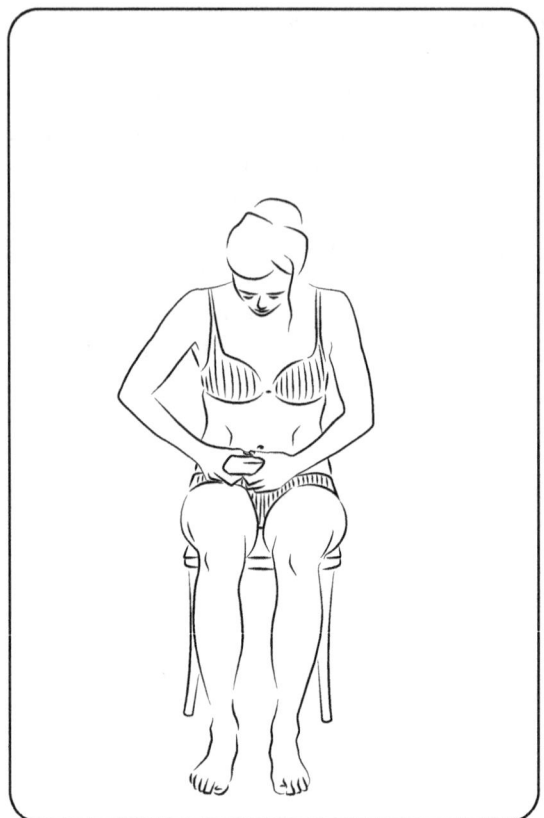

Fig. 4.13 Toilet Dance Exercise Starting Position

> Punktum mobile are the variations of movements that you can now perform. Make sure that you always stay with a certain movement sequence until the movement feels light and free and the pain or intensity has decreased by at least two thirds compared to the beginning.

Here are some proven examples of movement sequences during the toilet dance exercise

- Squats: Both feet including heels are (and remain) well in contact with the ground. Now start bending one knee while the other remains straight. Then bend the other knee while the other straightens again. The pelvis and hip on the respective side should tilt downwards. Continue this alternating movement until the tension decreases and you can stand up easily.

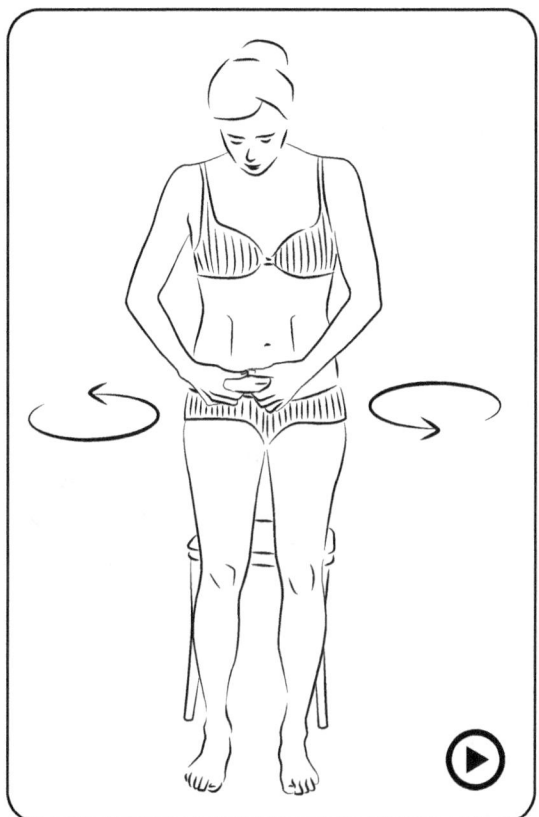

Fig. 4.14 Toilet Dance Exercise Execution. (© 2023 Liedler Concept ▶ https://doi.org/10.1007/000-fs4)

The exercise is finished when the feeling of tension under the hands has decreased by at least two-thirds compared to the beginning, you can stand upright easily and lightly, and the knee movement is smooth and tension-free.

- Pelvic circling: Circle your pelvis carefully and lovingly in one direction. The size of the circle is guided by the intensity of the tightness and the felt pull under your hands. Slowly and steadily, you increase the movement of the circle. The goal is for the pelvis to be able to circle maximally again, you can stand up well during this, and the intensity has decreased by at least two-thirds compared to the beginning. Afterwards, you can also circle the pelvis in the other direction.

- Walking in the room: Walk around the room with the scoop grip on your stomach. Strains of tension that now occur show you where and how adhesions affect every step. Continue walking until the stride length corresponds relaxed to your normal extent and you can walk relaxed despite the scoop grip. At the same time, the feeling of tension under the hands also subsides.

Afterwards, you can also try to increase the steps. Since this counts again as a new movement exercise, it is again important to complete it completely.

> **Important**
> - You control the intensity of the exercises through the speed and size of the movement of the Punktum mobile. The more carefully you approach the end of the range of motion to then slightly increase it, the more moderate and bearable are the intensity and pain during the entire self-exercise.
> - Always complete each exercise completely to end in a relaxed feeling of physical well-being!
> End = restored freedom of movement and reduced intensity by minus two-thirds

4.1.1.3.3 Stair Exercise

The stair exercise (see Figs. 4.15, 4.16 and 4.17) is primarily aimed at promoting the straightening and elongation of the longitudinal axis. The aim is to loosen the adhered tissue layers in this direction of movement in order to restore full freedom of movement.

> **Stair Exercise Instructions**
>
> The exercise always begins in a sitting position. Why? When sitting, the abdomen is relaxed and the adhesions can be easily grasped. With both hands, a part of the affected area or the scar is now encompassed along the longitudinal axis of the body with the scoop grip (fixed point) and fixed together with the affected tissue layers in depth.
>
> Then the hands are turned and the scoop grip is aligned perpendicular to the longitudinal axis of the body. To make this difficult hand position easier, I recommend bending over well and relaxing the abdomen. Then apply the scoop grip with one hand first and add the other hand twisted so that the thumbs of both hands are directed towards the head, one thumb on each side and the outer edge of the little fingers of both hands points towards the pelvis.

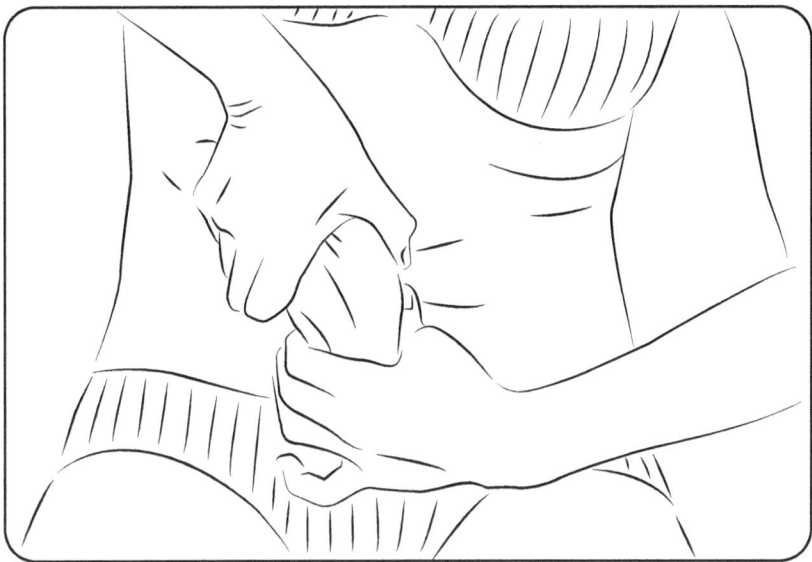

Fig. 4.15 Stair exercise hand position

With the correct scoop grip, an unpleasant to painful tension should now be felt in the targeted tissue and intensify as soon as you try to slowly straighten up. **Slowly**, as you do not yet know from when the adhesions really tense and possibly cause pain. You may not be able to straighten up completely at first. It is important that you dose the scoop grip and this initial tension so that you can keep it fixed throughout the entire LK self-exercise (fixed point).

The process always ends when the movement feels light and can be carried out widely. The intensity should decrease by at least two thirds compared to the beginning before the exercise is ended. From the starting position, you now add the following movements one after the other (mobile point as added movement):

- Alternate bending your knees. In doing so, the hip of the respective side always lowers as well. The heels remain in good contact with the ground throughout. Notice at the same time how your straightening improves.
- Circle your pelvis. First, circle it in one direction until it feels light and permeable. Then change to the other direction until the movement is also possible widely and lightly here. Also, pay attention to gradually straightening the upper body better.
- Walk around the room.
- Walk carefully step by step down stairs or downhill outdoors and feel any restrictions in the movement system. Continue the stair exercise until you can straighten up well and relaxed at the same time, the movement becomes smooth and light again and the perceived intensity or pain has decreased by at least two thirds.

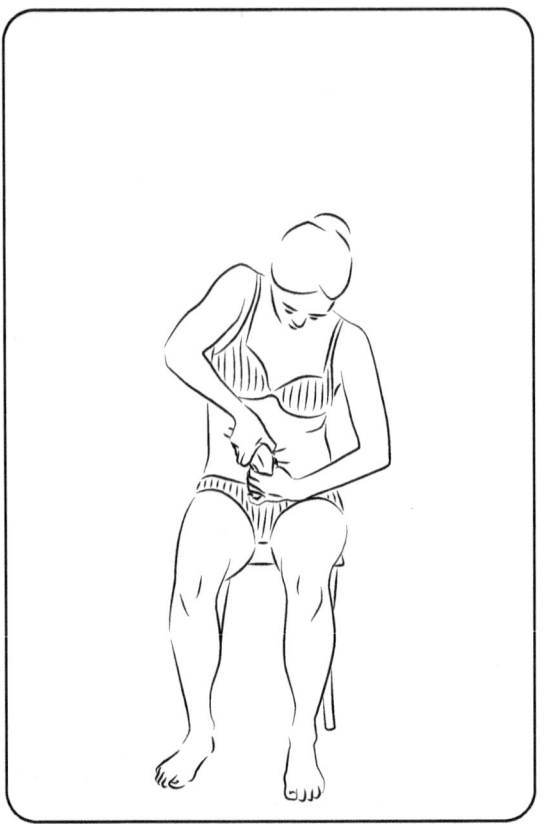

Fig. 4.16 Stair exercise starting position

4.1.1.3.4 Variations in Sitting, Standing, Walking

Once you feel confident with the prescribed exercises and the scoop grip, you can also try individual movement exercises at your own discretion: Create the fixed point with the scoop grip in the abdominal area or the affected area and test all movements for restrictions with the mobile point. Whether you tilt the pelvis, twist the upper body in various directions, circle the shoulders, hop or run. Any noticeable movement patterns can thus be tested and treated immediately. The important thing is always: If a movement is felt that triggers a feeling of tightness in the body or a pulling tension or pain, then stay mindful exactly with this movement, lovingly enlarge it as far as possible and always complete the exercise!

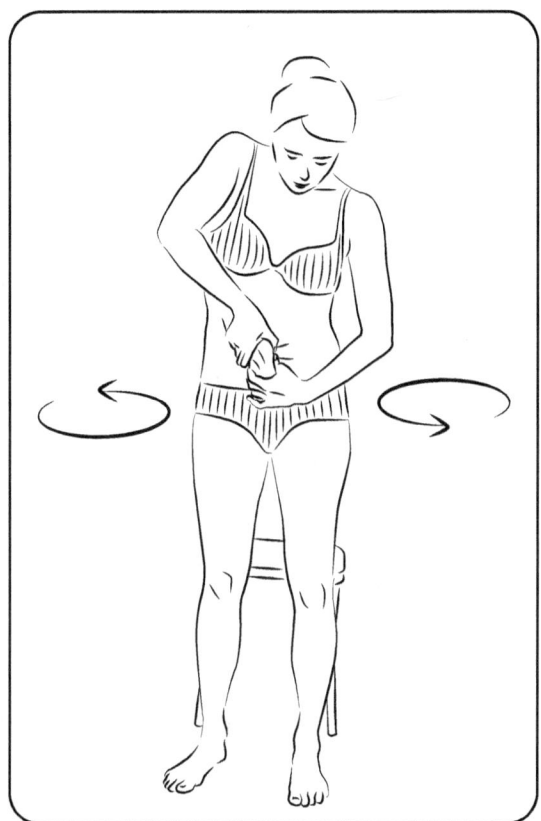

Fig. 4.17 Stair exercise execution

- Tilt, circle the pelvis
- Circle, lift, bend, stretch the hips
- Circle the shoulders
- Stretch, twist the upper body
- Walk, run, hop, lunge, dance step
- Dance
- Lift arm/s
- Twist, move, bend, stretch the spine

4.1.1.3.5 Variation for Other Body Parts

Every surgery always affects the superficial and deep tissue layers, which means that the LK self-exercises also promote mobility and body comfort in

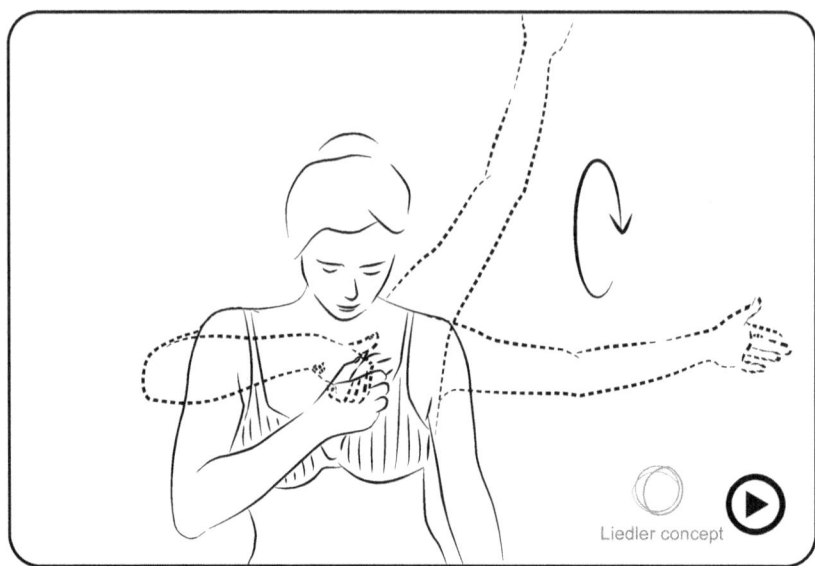

Fig. 4.18 Example of scar mobilization in the shoulder area. (@ 2022 Liedler-Concept. Individual Application—Example shoulder ▶ https://doi.org/10.1007/000-fs7)

surgeries beyond the abdominal area. In the LK self-exercises, the scar and its adhesions are related to the next larger joints, tested and treated if necessary (see Fig. 4.18).

Varying Starting Position (Creating the Fixed Point)
The starting position now varies individually depending on the surgery or scar. The LK focus and the LK principles remain the same. As does the procedure of the technique. Even if the scars on the surface are small, the scoop grip always refers to the potential iceberg below the scar in depth. This means that the scoop grip (fixed point) is always built up as large as possible and fixed with the largest possible fold, regardless of the externally visible scar.

Execution (Introducing the Mobile Point)
Depending on the area of surgery, the next larger joint is now moved through to its maximum freedom of movement. This can be the shoulder, the pelvis, the knee, the ankle joint, etc. Each joint normally has the ability to move relaxed and freely in different directions. How do you recognize what is "normal"? Here it is helpful that you have many of your joints double in the body. So if you are not sure how a joint "normally" moves, test the movement and the extent simply on the second joint. Based on this, you can now perform the technique of the mobile point. The technique is finished when, despite the scoop grip, the joint can move freely to its full extent and the intensity or painful sensation has decreased by at least two thirds compared to the beginning.

4.1.2 Aftereffects After Self-Treatment of Scars

Through the LK self-exercises changes of adhesions in the tissue and in the abdominal cavity and thus tissue remodeling processes are initiated. These real changes in the body are noticeable in the days following, depending on the intensity with which the exercises were performed. You must not forget that you are consciously creating a moderate inflammatory process so that the body can restructure the tissue. Even muscle soreness counts as such a reaction. The following after-reactions are therefore **normal** and should disappear within 2 to 7 days.

4.1.2.1 Physical and Mental After-Reactions

Scar therapy is strenuous. Through the triggered remodeling processes, however, a sustainable result is achieved. The gained sliding layers remain, existing and noticeable adhesions can always be further treated and resolved at any time.

What can such after-reactions look like in concrete terms?

Common

- Fatigue, feeling of exhaustion (1 to 2 days)
- Feeling of muscle soreness (1 to 4 days)
- Sore feeling and pulling in the treated or surrounding area (1 to 7 days)

Occasionally/Rarely

- Inner restlessness
- Emotional after-reaction—tears

4.1.2.2 Noticeable Positive Changes

The focus is of course on the improvements and reliefs that you want to achieve through the LK self-exercises. Make yourself actively aware of these! To be able to perceive the differences particularly well, it is helpful to direct your attention exactly to the part of the body where you can expect changes before the exercise. That means, if you are working on a specific area, pay close attention to where you can feel compactions, firmness or reduced elasticity. Your attention is primarily directed towards real tangible components of tissue such as hardness versus softness, restrictions in movements versus mobility, tension versus lightness, etc.

Any flexibility and mobility that increases in the tissue during the LK self-exercise means that the tissue is changing towards dynamic health. Each gained sliding layer means an increase in shiftability and suppleness and thus less tension in the affected area and subsequently in the rest of the body.

Direct your attention to the before and after: more and more elasticity, more and more ease in straightening your body and more and more smoother execution of movements. Movements that were previously accompanied by a pulling sensation gradually become tension-free. What previously manifested as a feeling of tightness in the body can transform layer by layer into space and freedom of movement.

Improvements through the treatment

- Better, easier straightening
- Feeling of lightness
- Feeling of losing ballast
- Improved mobility of the tissue in the scar area
- Improved deep shiftability of the tissue in the affected and surrounding scar area
- No more accompanying pulling in the tissue during stress or movement
- Decrease in chronic tension conditions (back, shoulder-neck, headaches, digestion…)
- Improvements in scar appearance

Even if our mind tends to focus attention primarily on existing tension, tension conditions or pain, the aim here is to sense and become aware of where it has actually become lighter and more supple in the body. Where has positive change taken place and what has become NEW?

4.1.2.3 Noticeable Changes in Breathing

Improved, deeper breathing into the abdomen

One area where breathing changes can be felt very clearly and quickly is the breath. Especially after abdominal surgeries, deep abdominal breathing is avoided for weeks due to the pain and is directed more into the chest.

The result is a protective posture, which in turn promotes the formation of adhesions in exactly those tissue layers that you actually need to move the abdomen well and loosely during breathing. Even if you consciously direct your breathing into your abdomen, it then feels impossible. The breathing remains shallow, which may lead to you repeatedly feeling like you're not getting enough air.

Working with the LK self-exercises leads to you regaining access to your deep breathing by restoring the sliding layers in the scar and iceberg area.

> **Mindful Breathing**
>
> Take a moment **before** performing the LK self-exercise and feel where and how your breath flows and expands in your body. Start by feeling the chest breathing. For this, place your hands on the front of your chest, on your sternum. Feel how your chest rises and falls with each breath. You may also feel how your shoulders rise and fall. Then place your hands on your upper abdomen and perceive how the breath shows there. Do you feel the expansion in all directions, forward, to the side, and backward? Then place your hands on your lower back. Do you feel an expansion there with the breath? Finally, make contact with your lower abdomen. Can you feel how your abdominal wall rises and expands with inhalation and sinks with exhalation? Or is the reverse breathing happening here? This means that you pull in your stomach with inhalation and push it out with exhalation. Observe and perceive. The aim is to create the conditions for you to consciously recognize changes.

After the LK self-exercises, relax again into your breathing and observe whether you can perceive changes. It may have become easier to direct the breath into the abdomen and to feel a breathing movement there. Do you feel like you can breathe deeper or get more air? Sometimes it takes a few practice rounds until enough tissue layers have been freed and there is enough space available again for a relaxed breathing movement.

> **Proper Breathing**
>
> Imagine your abdomen during breathing like a balloon: When you fill a balloon with air, it inflates, it becomes full and round. When you let the air out again, the balloon becomes narrow and flat. This means that with abdominal breathing, the abdomen is allowed to expand like a balloon with inhalation. With exhalation, the abdomen sinks in and the navel can be drawn towards the spine. It becomes flat, like a balloon from which the air escapes.

5

Questions and Answers

The consequences of surgeries are hidden invisibly under the skin. Neither the actual size of the wound deep within the body can be guessed, nor is it possible to see why something feels different than before or why something hurts. This can cause great uncertainty in the affected person. Also, because only a few doctors talk about possible after-effects and treatment options following surgery. Targeted scar therapies are rarely considered because the knowledge of their possible healing effect is not known. Instead, pain conditions and chronic tension after surgery are often attributed to the psyche and referred to as psychosomatic.

This part is dedicated to the most important questions that affected people ask and have asked in practice. Concrete answers should briefly and concisely facilitate the introduction to the topic of scars, support the implementation of LK self-exercises, or clarify any remaining open questions. A more detailed list of questions on this topic can be found at narbenzentrum.at or liedlertreatment4scars.com.

5.1 Questions about the Scar

5.1.1 When Does a Scar "Bother"?

There are different levels at which a scar can "bother". Basically, "bother" describes a state in which the scar is not peacefully and unobtrusively integrated into the body system, but the body still has to react to the scar after complete healing. What can bother on the mechanical level? Due to the reduced elasticity of the scar and adhesions in the tissue and in the abdomen the mobility is restricted. The body requires a permanent adjustment of the surrounding structures. Or there are excessive nerve impulses that constantly report back to the brain about the tissue changes in the scar area. Unrest can also arise on an emotional level: If the scar and the surgery are associated with traumatic experiences and fear, the affected body area often cannot be touched or is mentally suppressed. Both leave tension in the body system, which the body has to incorporate and balance into the entire system.

5.1.2 Do All Scars Bother?

Not all scars bother. If none of the above factors apply, the scar is white, inconspicuous, movable from the surface to the depth and freely dynamically movable, emotionally peaceful and neuronally inconspicuous. Then the scar is good and the interference field of the actual tissue changes on the surface—the scar—is minimal.

Small skin scars, such as those that occur after superficial wounds or abrasions or even after mole removals, often leave hardly a scar or such a minor impairment in the tissue that they form no or hardly any interference field.

5.1.3 Is There a Point in Time when a Scar Can No Longer Be Changed?

No. Regardless of the age of the scar, change in the tissue is always possible. The surgery and the formation of the scar as well as the adhesions had a point in time in the past. However, since the body constantly renews the tissue, the structures that make up the hardness in the tissue are always only a maximum of one and a half years old. Due to the constant adjustments and the corresponding remodeling of the body to the current influences, it is always and at any time possible to work with the tissue and change the information and thus the tissue there! This means to enhance suppleness and mobility instead of coming to terms with ongoing rigidity and firmness.

5.1.4 I Have No Complaints. Do I Need Scar Therapy at All?

If no complaints occur after surgery, then in the best case the body has healed the wound on the surface and also in the deep tissue layers well. What remains is only a minimal interference field, which the body can balance well. During the healing phase, the body reconnects the injured tissue layers with each other. This leads to the formation of adhesions in the tissue and in the depth of the abdominal cavity in the surgical area, which restrict sliding layers that can normally slide freely to each other. The movable tissue around this area now compensates for the resulting restrictions. If this works well, it may be that despite the scar and adhesion, no symptoms occur.

Nevertheless, it is always sensible to check with the LK scar test whether there are impairments when provoked. The effects might only show up years later when the body accumulates more tension in the further life story. With the LK scar test, it is possible to quickly and clearly make visible and noticeable whether and what effects the internal adhesion network has on the musculoskeletal system.

5.1.5 My Scar is Pulled Inward and Looks Like a Groove. I Have No Pain, but an Unpleasant Overhanging Tissue Fold Has Formed Above the Scar. Why is this?

An injury, e.g., a cesarean section, heals. To repair the cut and the opening of the injured tissue, the body must first pull together the wound edges and tissue layers to subsequently connect and glue them together. In the best case, the visible end product scar is then a fine, thin, white line. In addition, the wound extends internally to the depth of the abdominal cavity, in the case of a cesarean section to the uterus, in other operations to the desired area. During wound healing, this chain of connection between the layers also contracts into the depth. Since the external tissue around the scar is movable, the scar follows the firm pull inward towards the surgical field in the abdominal cavity. This becomes visible on the skin as a depression or groove. As with a belt that has been buckled too tightly, the supple soft abdominal tissue overlaps and bulges over the scar. This creates the overhanging tissue fold. Adhesions are often palpable and tangible as inelastic nodules, firm nodules, hardenings, or compactions under the skin.

5.1.6 The Scar is Still Numb after Several Years. Can Anything be Done about this?

In the course of the skin incision, fine nerves and pain receptors are injured, which the body then tries to repair. During the repair processes, compactions are formed, which can feel hardened and inelastic, which can change and prevent the sensitivity and stimulus conduction of the nerves. This can result in numbness. The better the original suppleness of the tissue can be restored, the more likely is also the return of normal sensitivity of the skin and tissue. At any time, consistent implementation of LK scar therapy helps until the tissue is soft and elastic again.

However, if skin nerves were really damaged during the surgery, it is still possible that a feeling of numbness remains despite movable tissue.

5.1.7 Is It True That You Should Not Massage the Scar because this Increases the Risk of Getting an Excessive Scar?

This is true as long as the wound edges are not well connected and healed. The issue is that tension, which pulls the wound edges apart during a massage, leads to delayed wound healing and a wider scar, and as a result, more scar tissue is deposited. However, once the scar is well closed and healed, it is indeed important to move and massage the scar tissue to restore suppleness! This also applies to the tissue layers below and around the scar, which often become firm and inelastic due to the surgery. The LK self-exercises are suitable for testing and treating these.

5.1.8 Six Months after My Cesarean Section, The Scar is Still Quite Red and Extremely Sensitive in Some Places. Should I Care for the Scar with Creams and Oils?

It is always good to keep the skin and the scar supple with creams. However, more relevant for the optimal interaction in the body is the restoration of the suppleness and mobility of the tissue layers to each other. This means: It is important to touch the scar and the scar area, to move the skin in all directions around the scar, and to shift the tissue layers. Wherever the tissue retracts or only moves with difficulty, adhesions are present. These should be softened through continuous movement and mobilization. Changes in sensitivity such as hypersensitivity, numbness, and redness indicate adhesions in the underlying, deeper tissue layers, as these restrictions poorly supply the tissue and can trigger nerve irritations. In addition, pain receptors grow into adhesions, which can massively influence the feeling of the skin due to the increased tension in the area. The moment the tissue is again elastic and movable, less tension is exerted on the nerves, the supply is improved, and the sensitivity can normalize again.

Deep tensions and adhesions after major surgery or a cesarean section should be tested and treated by an osteopath or physiotherapist in addition to the LK self-exercises, who specializes in the aftercare of scars and adhesions in the tissue and the abdominal cavity.

5.2 Questions about the LK Self-Exercises— Application

5.2.1 When is the Best Time to Treat the Scar with LK Self-Exercises?

It is important to deal with the scar from the beginning. Every surgery represents an intervention and a permanent change of the skin surface and deep tissue layers. Once the wound is well closed and the crust has fallen off, one can already begin to gently support the body in restoring the sliding layers in the scar area. As soon as the treating doctor has given the go-ahead for sports, work can also begin on the adhesions in the deep layers. Since the body progressively optimizes and improves the affected area throughout the first year after the surgery, it is advisable to start with the LK self-exercises immediately after the surgeon's clearance to prevent protective postures and further tensions in the body.

Basically, the body always reorganizes itself, depending on the impulses and stresses it is exposed to. This also applies to scar tissue. This means, it is never too late to start therapy and the self-exercises.

5.2.2 How Often Do I Have to Do the LK Self-Exercises Until I Can Feel Improvements?

A daily application is recommended. The LK self-exercises are designed to fit well into everyday life and can also be applied as needed. With proper execution, you will notice relief in the affected area and also in the rest of the body after each treatment. Each application breaks down adhesions and restores the sliding of tissue layers. The more frequently and intensively you apply the exercises, the more noticeable and faster you will feel changes. However, I ask you to be patient. Since during an surgery both the skin is opened and the tissue is injured far into the depth of the body space, this means that many tissue layers and sliding layers are affected by the adhesions. Each one counts. This means, the more layers you treat with the LK self-exercises, the better and lighter you will feel.

5.2.3 Over What Period of Time Do I Have to Treat the Scar?

My recommendation is to treat the scar and the adhesions as long as you feel comfortable again in your body and with your scar, the movement layers are freely movable and you have regained the feeling of inner space and width. As long as the scar can trigger pulling feelings, there is definitely still a need for treatment. Tension states should have decreased or disappeared completely and the scar may become calmly inconspicuous.

5.2.4 Why Does Scar Therapy Have to Hurt? Are There also Pain-Free Variants?

In the healing process of a wound, altered tissue structures are formed, which lose their mobility and are often rigid, dense and immobile. In the area of the scar, they can be felt as hard strands or knots or lumps. Pain sensors grow into these densifications of the scar and adhesions, which normally lie loosely in the movable tissue. If stimuli such as tension or pressure act on the scar and adhesions, these pain sensors are activated more easily and trigger a pain stimulus. The more careful you apply the techniques, the less discomfort or pain you feel.

The aim of scar therapy is to stimulate the body to rebuild the adhesions into movable structures. Therefore, in LK scar therapy, we work directly with these dense structures that cause pain easily, in order to trigger a stimulus exactly there. We make use of the feedback from the sensors in scar therapy, as it indicates where and how many adhesions can be found in this area. The felt tension, discomfort or pain during the LK self-exercises can always be dosed and controlled and is ALWAYS BEARABLE if the LK technique is performed correctly. At the same time, the decrease in discomfort or pain during treatment can be used to track how the adhesions are loosening and the tissue is becoming supple and soft again.

5.2.5 Can the Scar Tear Open again Through the LK Self-Exercises?

No, with the correct application of LK scar therapy, it is not possible to tear open the scar or the tissue again. The intensity is always chosen with great care both in therapy and in LK self-application, thereby respecting the load limit of the tissue. The aim is to send impulses into the tissue, in response to which the body then reacts with its own adequate remodeling processes.

5.2.6 What Does It Mean if the Skin Directly at the Cesarean Section Scar Cannot be Lifted at all? What Do I Do Then?

A scar that cannot be lifted at all indicates that it is very tightly and fixedly adhered to the deeper underlying tissue layers. Ideally, the scar should be soft and easily movable and shift from the surface to the depth.

Here it helps to imagine the image of an iceberg during the LK self-exercises: The superficial scar represents the tip of the iceberg, the adhesions the much larger part of the iceberg in the depth of the tissue. If you want to treat a scar that cannot be lifted, then you must assume that the iceberg extends far beyond the visible scar field. If you now apply the technique in the iceberg area, i.e. where you can lift a fold with the scoop grip, then you achieve a positive effect on this entire area including the scar. Additionally, it helps, for example, to lean the upper body forward while sitting to also reduce the tension in the abdominal area in order to better grip the folds with the scoop grip.

5.2.7 How Should I Grip during the LK Self-Exercises? Do I Always Place My Hands Along the Scar on the Skin?

A scar is good when it can be moved and lifted freely in all directions. This also means for the LK self-exercises that the fold can be formed with the scoop grip in all directions. In the beginning, it makes sense to form and lift the fold in the direction that is possible. This can be along the scar, but also across or diagonally. It is important that you can hold it well throughout the entire LK self-exercise. Here it is advisable to choose the fold rather too large than too small. The adhesions under the skin otherwise easily pull the gripped fold out of your fingers.

5.2.8 After a Period of Positive Change, My Body Feels the Same as before. Have the Adhesions Come Back?

No, that is not the case. Everything that is resolved is kept in motion through everyday life and sports. The body becomes more supple, which also affects the movements. Often, things and movements are then automatically done again, running, hiking, stretching further than was possible in the tight state before. As these movement possibilities increase, the body's limits are stressed anew and it may be that a "new end of flexibility" appears. This end usually shows itself in the well-known symptoms. It seems as if nothing has changed and everything has come back. However, it merely means that there is a new layer of movement in the depth that was not demanded and moved in this form before and indicates adhesions that now needs to be resolved. These adhesions were well fixed by the outer adhesions until now and therefore not/ hardly noticeable. Normally, it is indeed the case that the body now shows the next layers where it needs help and support to resolve them and further exploit the range of motion.

5.3 Preparation for an Operation, Support of Wound Healing and Therapy

5.3.1 How and What Can I Contribute to Ensure that the Scar Heals Nicely?

It is important for a nice scar that as little tension as possible is exerted on the scar edges and pulls them apart. The more the scar is pulled apart in the first weeks, the more likely it is to form a rather wide scar. Special silicone patches can support the scar in healing as tension-free as possible.

To promote the suppleness of the scar, the scar can additionally be treated with shifts and light massages, if the crust has fallen off and the scar is closed and healed.

Also, special ointments, St. John's wort oil or scar oils with anti-inflammatory components help to support the subsiding inflammatory processes.

5.3.2 How Can I Additionally Support Wound Healing?

Basically, the more relaxed you go through the process of the surgery, the better for the subsequent wound healing. This includes on a physical level that you are as flexible as possible and the wound healing can thus take place in a flexible environment. This helps to prevent adhesions.

Body therapists, osteopaths, physiotherapists or certified LK therapists can support you in this.

Relaxation promotes a good wound healing process. Pay close attention to yourself, your limits and needs in the first days and weeks after the surgery. Be loving and mindful with yourself, listen to the signals of your body, allow yourself breaks when you need them. Everything is allowed that feels good and leaves a greater sense of well-being in the body afterwards.

Good and basic alkaline food can also contribute to reducing inflammation more quickly.

GPSR Compliance

The European Union's (EU) General Product Safety Regulation (GPSR) is a set of rules that requires consumer products to be safe and our obligations to ensure this.

If you have any concerns about our products, you can contact us on

ProductSafety@springernature.com

In case Publisher is established outside the EU, the EU authorized representative is:

Springer Nature Customer Service Center GmbH
Europaplatz 3
69115 Heidelberg, Germany

www.ingramcontent.com/pod-product-compliance
Lightning Source LLC
LaVergne TN
LVHW010344260326
834688LV00036B/870